Abs and Back

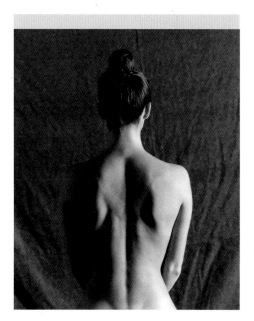

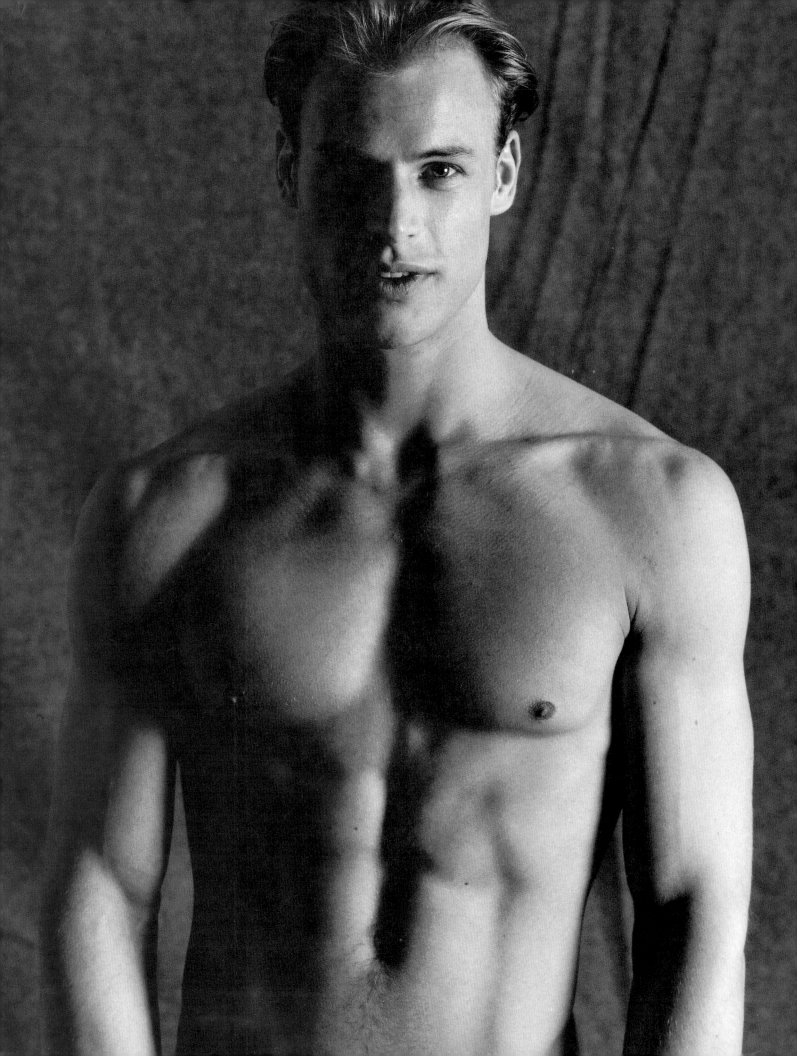

The Supple Workout

Abs and Back

Mark Bender

Photography by Antonia Deutsch

MACMILLAN • USA

MACMILLAN
A Simon and Schuster Macmillan Company
1633 Broadway
New York, NY 10019

A DBP Book
conceived, created and designed by
Duncan Baird Publishers
Sixth Floor
Castle House
75-76 Wells Street
London W1P 3RE

A catalogue record is available from the Library
of Congress.
ISBN 0-02-861344-9

Designers: Sue Bush, Gail Jones
Editor: Stephanie Driver
Commissioned Photography: Antonia Deutsch

10 9 8 7 6 5 4 3 2 1

Typeset in Frutiger
Colour reproduction by Bright Arts, Hong Kong
Printed in Singapore

Publishers' note
The exercises in this book are intended for
healthy people who want to be fitter. However,
exercise in inappropriate circumstances can be
harmful, and even fit, healthy people can injure
themselves. The publishers, DBP, the author, and
the photographer cannot accept any
responsibility for any injuries or damage incurred
as a result of using this book.

Contents

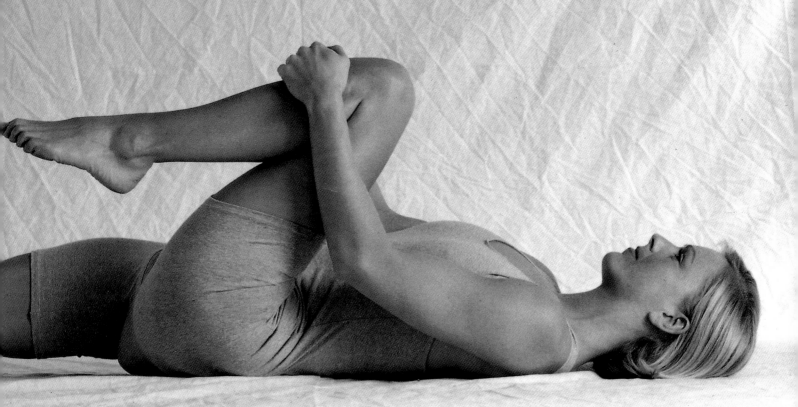

Introduction

Each body is unique. We all have different strengths and weaknesses, but all too often we dwell on our weaknesses and fail to recognize our strengths and how useful these strengths could be in realizing our full potential – if we only took the trouble to explore what is possible.

The exercises in this book will teach you how to improve the condition of your abs and your back. This will lead not only to an enhanced appearance, as you stand straighter and your midriff is firmer, but you will also feel a great sense of well-being, as you breathe deeply and fully and feel the strength of your new, more dynamic body.

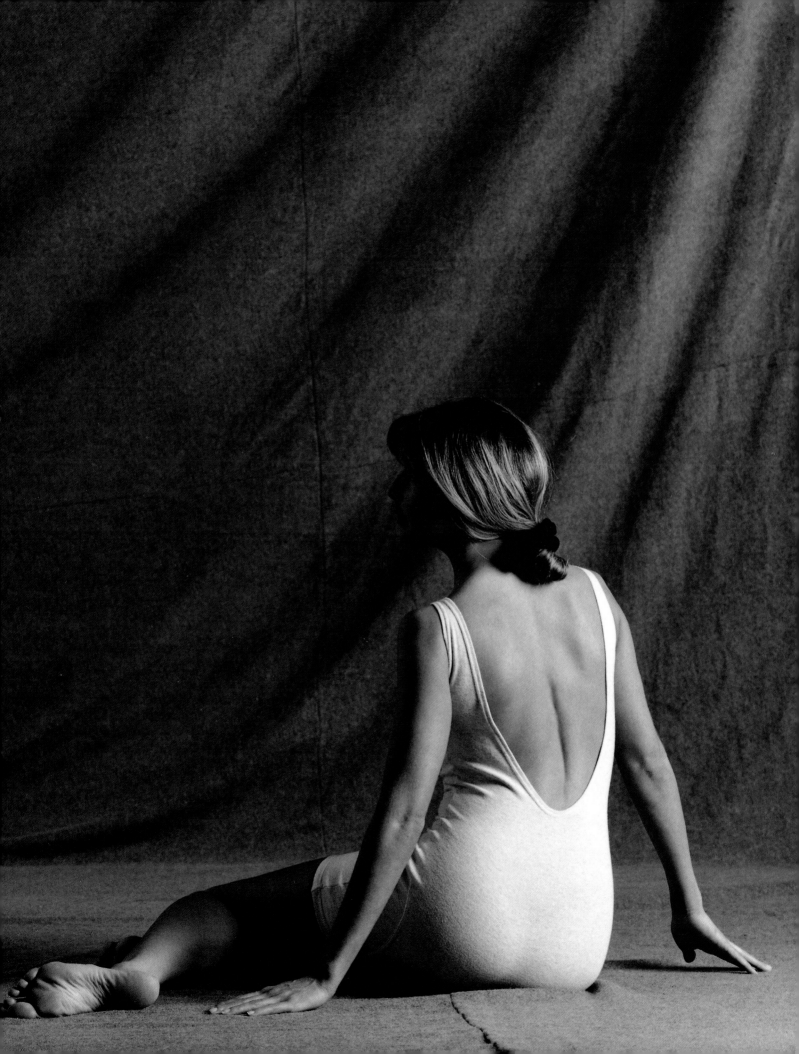

Getting started:
how to use this book

The exercises in this book have been designed so they do not require a major time commitment and so they can be done anywhere or anytime. You do not need any special equipment or clothing.

Success – improvement in your posture and relief of any back aches and pains – will be quicker if you integrate the Core Exercises with some of the exercises from the Total Body Workout section.

For best results, do the exercises little and often every day. A total of 10 minutes exercise three to four times a day is ideal. You may even want to repeat your favorite exercises each hour, particularly at first. This will make you more aware of your posture and improve the endurance of those muscles that hold you upright against gravity.

Remember, the most effective exercises for your abs and back are not the ones that make you sweat and strain. Work slowly and carefully, taking the time to listen to your body and learn to understand the way your abdominal and back muscles function.

You do not need a separate warm-up before beginning the Core Exercises or the Total Body Workout, but remember to work gently at the start of your exercise until your muscles begin to feel free.

The exercises in this book are safe if you follow the instructions correctly. However, if you have persistent lower back pain, consult your physician immediately. If you have severe spinal problems, it is best to consult your physical therapist or your physician before beginning any exercise program.

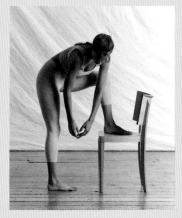

Core exercises, pages 22–43
Focusing on the abdominals and the back, these exercises will stretch and strengthen the muscles of your torso, helping you to develop a more vibrant and upright appearance and a healthier spine.

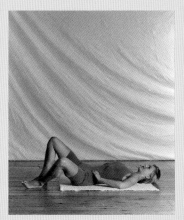

Warm-ups, pages 44–53
Before you begin any vigorous activity, such as playing a sport or doing work around the house, it is important to warm up the body. These exercises will prepare the muscles of your lower back and stomach to support your body.

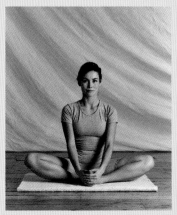

Total body workout, pages 54–67
These exercises are designed to increase the stability of your trunk and pelvis by working the muscles of your lower back, your abdominals, and your buttocks. Stronger muscles in the trunk and the pelvis will help the body to move more efficiently, lessening strain on the spine.

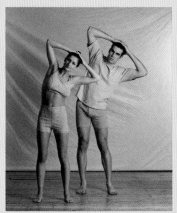

Routines, pages 68–77
It is easy to fit exercise into any lifestyle. Here are two examples of routines tailored for specific circumstances. Pause Gymnastics are exercises designed to be done regularly when you are working at a desk, in order to avoid strain in your back and arms. The Home Energizer exercises are perfect for people who do not play sports but want some simple but dynamic exercises to do at home.

Back to basics:
posture

Take some time to remember the basics. If you treat your back without respect, sitting badly and straining as you lift heavy objects, there is a good chance you will pay the price. However, by remembering a few simple rules and doing a few easy exercises every day, your back will not only stay supple and relaxed, but your body will look great. And the really good news is that it couldn't be easier.

Nearly every movement you make – sitting down in a chair, walking to the front door, bending down to tie your shoe or to turn on the TV – involves your back in one way or another. Despite this, far too many of us take the workings of the back, and particularly the spine, for granted.

The back is also the key to a healthy posture. Posture is one of the main means by which we present ourselves to the world. For example, a depressed person will often appear bent or slouched, while a captain of industry will demand respect and obedience by puffing out his chest and holding his back ram-rod straight. An older actress will tell you that she can carry on playing youthful parts on stage by keeping her back supple, because the hunched back is perhaps the single biggest sign of ageing.

At the same time, posture is very closely linked to our emotional state, as well as our physical one. Our emotional state has two components: one is purely mental, and the other is physiological, and these two interact. The mind may instruct the body to respond in a particular way: for example, when we feel emotional pain, we often contract our body as if to protect it from harm. However, the mind also analyzes the state of the body and draws conclusions: if we sit and stand in a slouched position, the mind may interpret this as insecurity. Therefore, as you improve your posture, you will begin to feel more dynamic and more secure – this is why working on your back is such a rewarding experience.

A healthy posture not only looks and feels positive, but it also allows the body to function in an optimal way. Unfortunately there is much bad advice available when it comes to physical posture, and it is easy to forget that a healthy posture is the most natural thing in the world. Remember this as you work through the routines in this book.

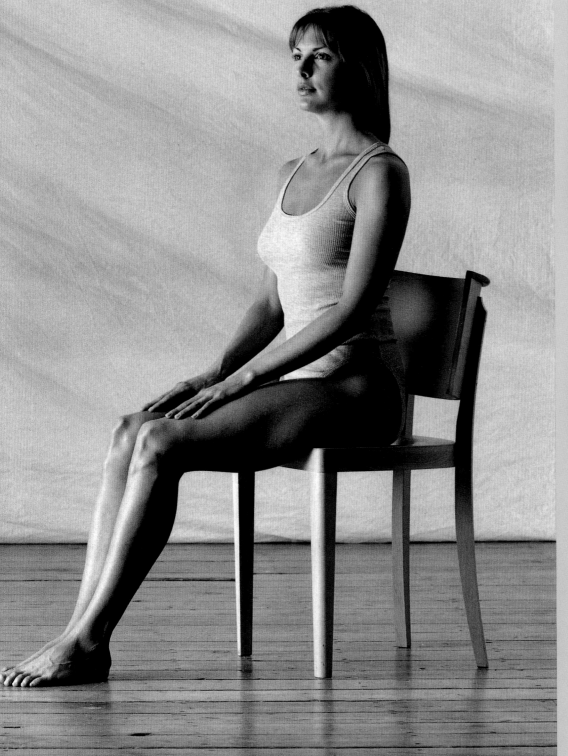

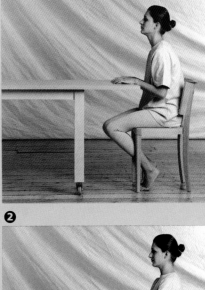

Sitting

Sitting slouched, with your chin jutting out, strains your back (1). To sit correctly (2), ensure that the height of your chair and desk are adjusted to your body size. Your feet should be flat on the floor, with your thighs not quite parallel to the floor. Your forearms should be parallel to your work surface.

The best way to understand how relaxed and resourceful the physical body can be is to look at the body of a child. A young child's back is long and straight, yet it is still relaxed. The head is balanced at the top of the spine without any unnecessary tension. Obviously everyone will lose some flexibility with age, but at the same time, many of us make physical activity harder than it needs to be. Much of the advice that is given here was second nature to us when we were children.

Sadly, we soon lose the child's easy, natural posture. Long hours are spent sitting in front of a computer screen or TV. We drive to the store instead of walking, and we stop playing sports once we leave school. All these factors, combined with the stress and strain of everyday living in the modern world, take their toll. Consequently you may find that your back feels stiffer than it used to, or in some cases you may find that the combination of poor posture and inactivity has led to spinal pain and muscular injury.

Think about your normal position when you sit. Do you slouch, with your chest concave and your bottom toward the front of the chair? This puts undue stress on the spinal disks and ligaments, and your back muscles and abdominals cannot support the spine. And if your head is thrust forward, this puts strain on your upper neck, often resulting in arm pains and headaches. A correct sitting posture will not create any unnecessary tension in the body. However, it is not a relaxed state either. Your lower back muscles should be working to keep your spine erect.

When you sit or stand with incorrect posture, you also restrict your breathing. The lungs have no muscles of their own: they take in air as they respond to changes in the size of the chest cavity created by movements of the muscles around the ribs, the back, and the abdomen. If you are slouched, the amount of space available for your lungs to expand is limited. As soon as the muscles in this part of the body are aligned and allowed to move freely, you will begin naturally to take deeper, more satisfying breaths.

To set yourself back on the road to that healthy state, you must begin to become more aware of how the back works. But remember, the aim is to release your back, allowing you to recognize its full potential. This cannot be forced or hurried. Simply telling yourself to

❶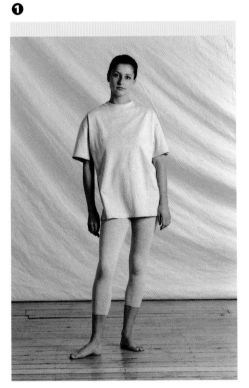

❷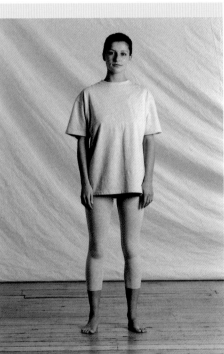

Standing

Standing with your weight over one hip, and your back and neck unaligned, not only looks unattractive, but can also lead to discomfort (1). When you are standing with good posture (2), your weight is evenly divided over both legs. Ideally, your whole body, from your ears through your shoulders, hips, and knees to your ankles, should be in alignment. Your knees and feet should be parallel and facing forward, with your weight balanced over your entire foot. Your abdominal muscles should be gently pulled in and up, supporting your lower back in its natural curve. Your shoulders should be parallel to the floor. Your head should be resting lightly on your neck, so your chin neither juts forward nor tucks down.

stand up straight or forcing your shoulders to relax will certainly do more harm than good. Excessive tension is the enemy of a healthy posture. However, as your muscles grow stronger and more accustomed to working together in a dynamic fashion, your posture will improve naturally.

Begin by trying this experiment. Sit on a firm chair and rest your hands on your thighs. Do nothing for a moment – just breathe easily and allow yourself to relax. Begin to picture your spine in your mind's eye (see the diagram on page 20 for reference). Take the index finger of your left hand and rest it as far down toward the bottom of your spine as possible. This will be about the top of your buttocks. Then, take the index finger of your right hand and rest it as high up your spine as possible. This will be just beneath the back of your skull between your ears. The distance from one finger to the other is the length of your spine. Long, isn't it?

Keeping your fingers where they are, experiment by moving your back in various ways. Slouch as much as possible, then sit up straight. Bend sideways or try to move only isolated parts of the spine. Notice whether

different positions have any effect on your breathing. This will help you become more aware of the range of movement of which your spine is capable, and the more you become aware of this, the more that range of movement will increase.

By doing the exercises in this book, you will learn to be more aware of your posture. In addition, as your abdominal and back muscles grow stronger, your posture will improve without your making any conscious effort.

As you work through this book, then, you will begin to feel the benefits of having a stronger and more supple back and torso. You will feel taller, looking life straight in the eye.

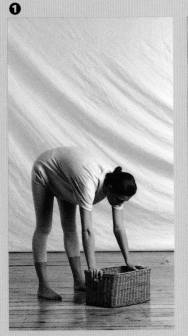
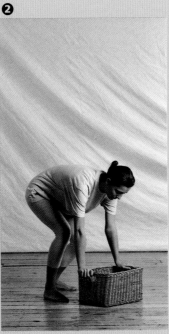
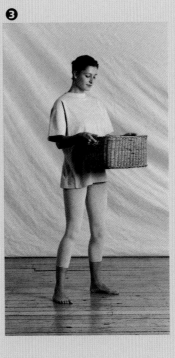
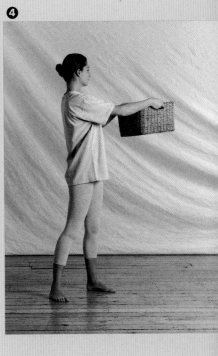

Lifting

Lifting heavy objects with your knees locked straight and bending from the waist can lead to serious injury (1). Good lifting technique (2) means getting close to the object you are about to lift and bending your knees rather than your back. Feet should be wide apart to give you a good base of support. Always lift with your knees bent, keeping your back straight. It may be safer to "pre-set" your abs, tensing your lower abdominal muscles and lifting the object as you breathe out. When you are carrying heavy objects, keep them close to your body, to avoid strain on your shoulders, but do not lean backward (3). Do not twist your body as you are lifting – this combination of bending and twisting is responsible for more spinal injuries than any other form of movement. Rather, turn your body once you are standing straight (4). If you are going to be doing heavy lifting or other physical work, do a few warm-up exercises first.

Body facts

The human body is an intricate construction, with an amazing range of movement. Even the simplest movement is the result of a complex interaction of bone, muscle, connective tissue, and nervous system.

The spine, in particular, is a triumph of natural engineering. It consists of 24 oddly-shaped bones, formed so as to allow a remarkable range of movement – as long as the supporting muscles, in the back and abdomen, are strong and supple.

In order to improve the condition of your abs and back, you should understand the ways in which the muscles work together.

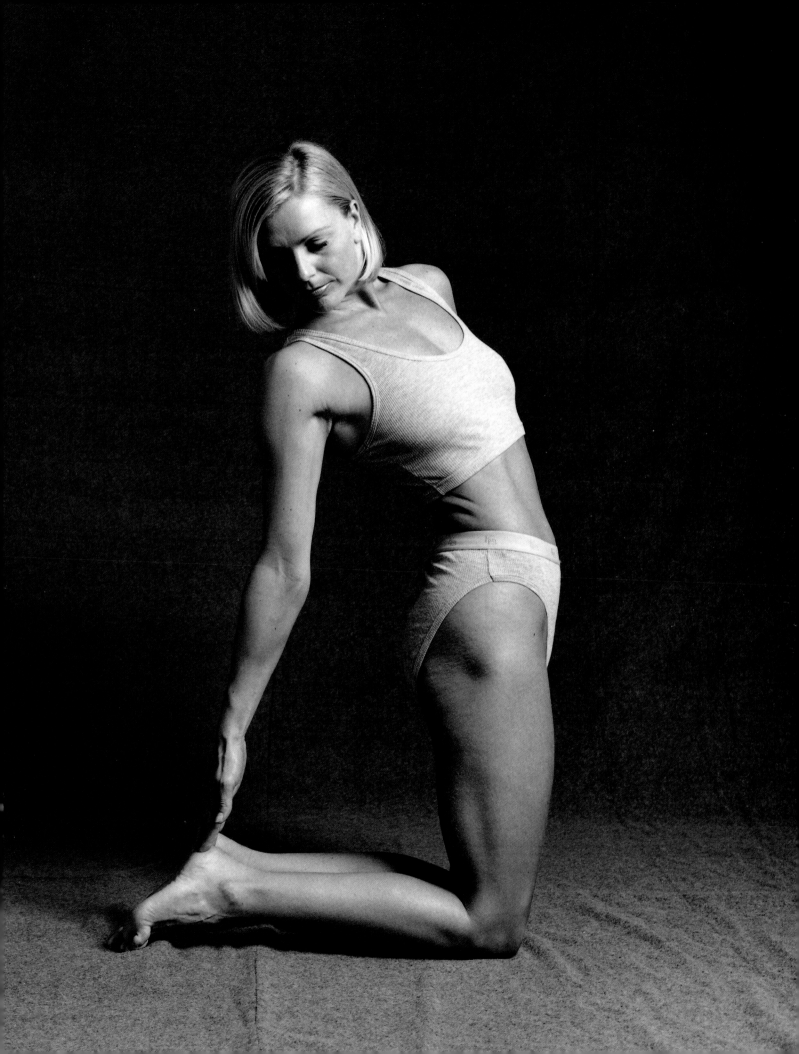

Body facts: abs and back

The torso – the back, abdomen, and chest – is the platform around which the arms and legs move. The trunk must be stable enough to support this movement and to stand upright, but it must also allow a wide range of motion, so you can bend forward and reach up and backward.

The spinal column is the foundation for the muscles of the back and neck. The vertebrae have different shapes and sizes depending on which part of the spine they come from. Those making up the lower back have wide, thick bodies, so they can cope with the forces coming down from the arms and upper back. The lower spine is designed to move backward and forward.

The 12 vertebrae that make up the mid-back, or thoracic spine, have special features to allow more twisting, or rotation, to occur. They also form joints with the ribs, which pass from the sides of the thoracic vertebrae around to the front of the chest where they form more joints with the chest bone. The neck is above the thoracic spine. It is designed to allow a great amount of movement and flexibility in all directions.

The pelvis is the basin on which the spinal column sits, and it connects the trunk to the legs. The stability of the pelvis allows the spine and legs to transmit forces through it.

The muscles that pass around the spine are responsible for both the dynamic stability of the spine and its movement. Each muscle has a specific function, and they all work in partnership to hold the body upright against gravity and to allow complex movements.

The muscles that aid the dynamic stability in the spine are deep muscles, lying very close to the disks and the vertebral bodies. Some pass over just one joint, but others may pass five or six different vertebral levels, with attachments to each vertebra. The muscles closer to the surface are moving muscles. Further muscles around the mid-back fix the shoulder blades to the spine and are responsible for both the mobility of the shoulders and arms.

The muscles at the front of the chest work in opposition to the back muscles to keep the spinal cord balanced. If there were no muscles at the front of the chest, the muscles of the back would pull the spinal cord backward.

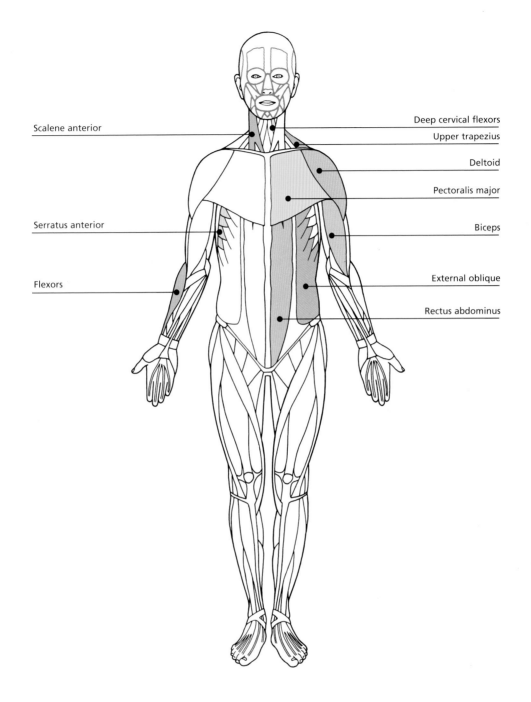

Scalene anterior

Deep cervical flexors

Upper trapezius

Deltoid

Pectoralis major

Serratus anterior

Biceps

Flexors

External oblique

Rectus abdominus

Front of the body

The abdominals are a group of four different muscles. One, the rectus abdominus, runs upward on either side of the midline of the body, from the pubic bone to the ribs. Its rippled form is easy to see on lean, highly developed bodies. The other three abdominals are flat sheets, layered one on top of the other. Underneath the external oblique are the internal oblique and the transverse abdominus. The muscles of the chest and shoulders work in opposition to the upper back muscles. If the chest is tight, the shoulders and upper back will hunch.

Cervical spine
- neck pain
- headaches
- arm pain

Listed on the left, under the relevant headings, are regions of the body in which discomfort can be caused by problems in particular areas of the spine.

The muscles of the lower back also cross the pelvis and literally anchor the spinal column to the pelvis. They are responsible for keeping the whole spine in a balanced position.

The abdominal muscles work in unison with the lower back muscles and the muscles around the pelvis to keep this main platform stable. The abdominal muscles closest to the surface act as movement muscles, bending the trunk forward. The deeper abdominal muscles stabilize the lower back.

The buttock muscles pass across the lower back and pelvis. They keep the hip and lower leg in alignment with the spinal column, and act as the main propulsive force of the body when walking or running. At the same level but to the front of the spine are the hip flexors. These originate from the front of the vertebrae and pass through the pelvis to exit onto the top of the leg. They bend the leg forward and stabilize the lower back.

Because of the way in which the muscles of the body interact, problems in one area of the back may cause discomfort in other parts of the body (see illustration, right).

Thoracic spine
- shoulder pain
- upper back pain
- neck pain

Lumbar spine
- lower back pain
- groin pain
- thigh/calf pain

Sacrum spine
- lower back pain
- leg pain

The spine
The spine is made up of 24 vertebrae, which are like bony building blocks stacked on top of each other. They are linked by two projections of bone at the back of each vertebra, one facing up and one down. The point at which these projections connect is a facet joint, and this is where movement in the spine occurs. This movement is limited by the contour of the bones – when they contact each other, further movement is blocked. The vertebrae are separated from each other by disks. They act as shock absorbers for the forces going up and down the spine and as a base on which each vertebra can pivot.

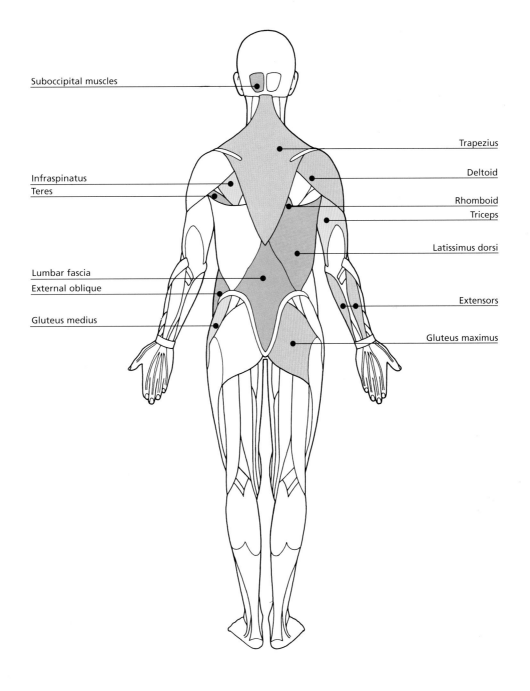

Suboccipital muscles

Infraspinatus
Teres

Lumbar fascia
External oblique

Gluteus medius

Trapezius

Deltoid

Rhomboid
Triceps

Latissimus dorsi

Extensors

Gluteus maximus

Back of the body

The muscles that aid the dynamic stability of the spine are very deep, lying close to the vertebrae. The muscles that are closer to the surface are the ones that are involved in movement. The external obliques are part of the abdominal group, which wrap nearly all the way around the body. The gluteus maximus is the major muscle of the buttocks: the condition of this muscle gives the buttocks their shape. The shoulder muscles, an intricate group, attach to the shoulder blades and to the collar bone. They work in opposition to the chest muscles.

Core exercises

If you spend a lot of time sitting during the day, the muscle groups running from the pelvis to the head will become progressively weaker with age. As these muscles struggle to hold your spine erect against the force of gravity, the joints of the spine become stiffer.

These core exercises will improve the strength of the supporting spinal muscles and the flexibility of the spine. Having a healthy spine will keep you looking and feeling younger and stronger. You will also feel healthier and more aware of your body when you do these exercises on a regular basis.

We all have different weak areas in our spines, so you can choose to focus on your own areas of discomfort. But if you are free of aches and pain, choose two or three exercises from each of the four sections. A few minutes' daily practice will allow you to maintain a strong and supple spine.

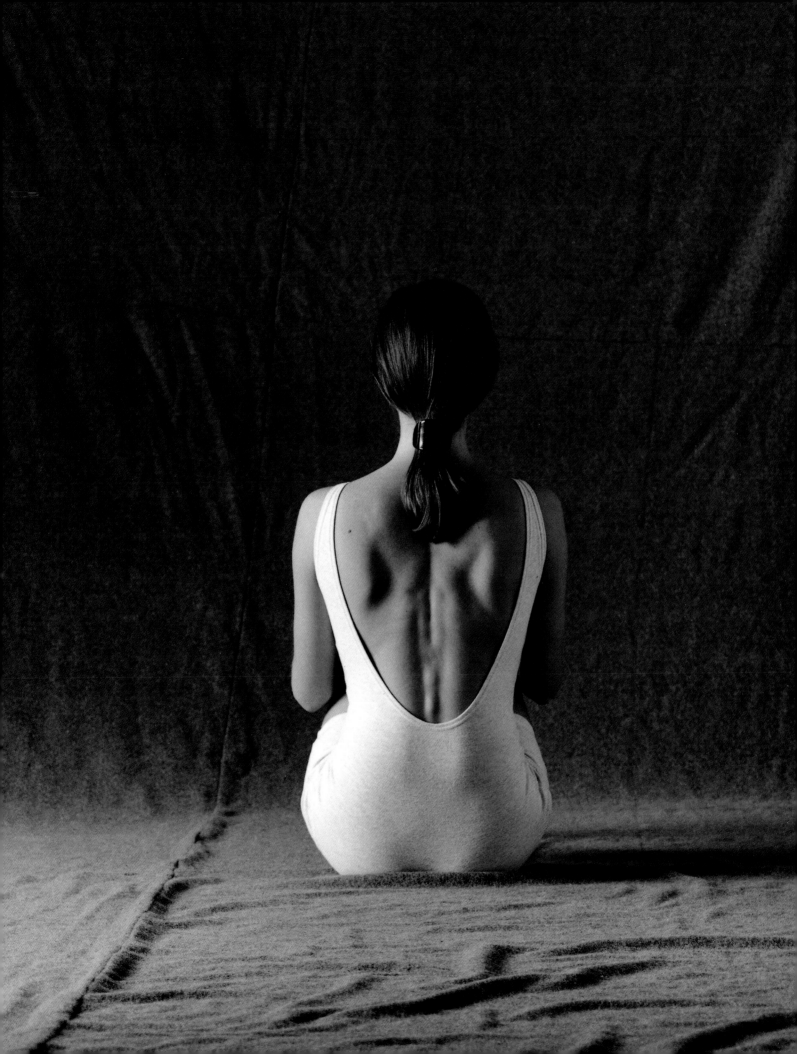

Head and neck

The group of muscles lying deep at the front of your neck is responsible for holding your head in good alignment on top of your spine and shoulders. If you sit with your head poking forward, these muscles weaken, and the muscles at the base of your skull tighten. When this happens, you feel an ache and stiffness at the top of your spine, and you may even experience headaches as the joints at the top of your neck take too much strain.

With exercises for the neck, it is essential to work gently. You should not feel any pain, and as soon as you feel you are losing control of what you are doing during an exercise, you must stop. Even if you can only do four or five repetitions of each exercise, this is enough. It is better to start slowly, gradually increasing the endurance of the muscles: if you push yourself too fast at the beginning, you can strain your neck muscles.

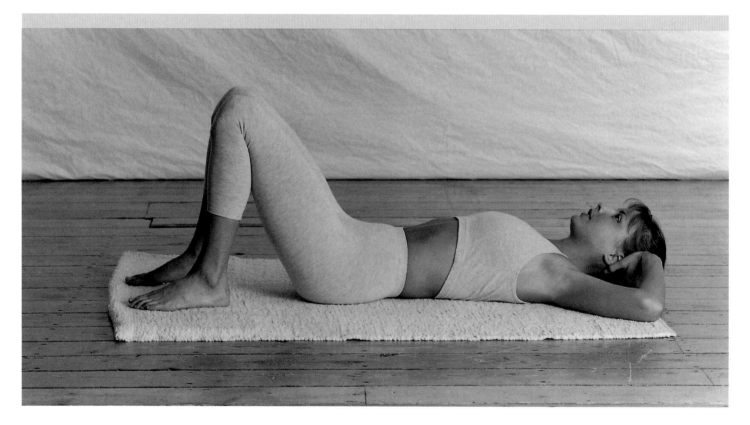

Neck lengthener

This exercise relaxes the muscles at the base of your skull, freeing them from tension caused by your daytime posture. It is also a good introduction to the other neck exercises.

Lying on your back (with your head on a pillow if you want), bend your knees and place your feet flat on the floor. Breathing slowly, deeply, and rhythmically, reach up with your hands and place your fingertips into the hollow between your neck and your skull. Gently press your fingers into the muscle, and use your hands to lengthen your neck. As you do this, your chin should naturally tuck in. Hold this pressure firmly but without strain for 30 seconds to one minute. Repeat the exercise rhythmically for two to three minutes in total.

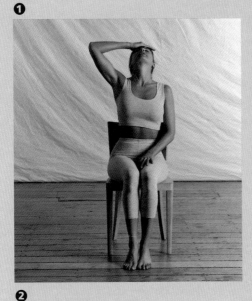

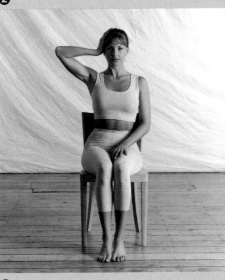

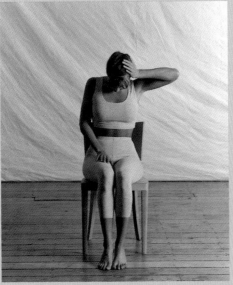

Head control series

This series of exercises is designed to strengthen the long muscles going from your shoulders to your neck and head. They are found at the front, back, and side of your neck.

Sitting tall, with your head balanced naturally on your neck, place both your hands on your forehead and apply pressure with your hands as if you were going to push your head backward. You should match this pressure from your hands with an equal pressure from the muscles around your neck, keeping your head in the mid-position – don't allow your hands to move your head. Start off gently, and gradually increase the pressure from your hands.

This exercise should be done gently and should be pain-free. You can vary the position of your head, applying the pressure to the front, back, and sides of your head, either with your head flopped forward, chin on your chest, or while looking up toward the ceiling, so your head is arching backward. For example, placing your hand on your forehead and tipping your head gently back, you can push forward with your head as you push lightly back with your hand (1). Or place your right hand on the right side of your head, just above your ear. Apply pressure with your hand, trying to push your head to your left shoulder (2). Again, don't let this movement happen: resist it with the muscles around your neck. You can do the same thing while your head is in a forward position (3).

Upper back

Your upper back stores a lot of tension, especially if you spend time sitting at a desk or working at a computer. In addition, when you feel stress, this part of your body tightens: just talking about being "uptight" can make your shoulders rise toward your ears.

The muscles of the upper back need to be both strong and supple: strong enough to contribute to the stability of the torso, and supple enough to allow the spine its full range of twisting movement, in order to prevent strain on the shoulder joints and the neck.

Some of these exercises will stretch the upper back and spine, and others will make the muscles around the upper back and shoulders work more efficiently. Decide which you are in need of most – more movement or more strength – and make your choice of exercises accordingly.

Even if you have a forward curve in this part of your back and you haven't been able to straighten up for some time, you will notice changes occurring quickly as you start to move in a healthier way.

❶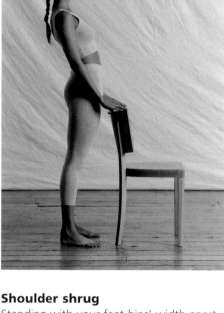

❷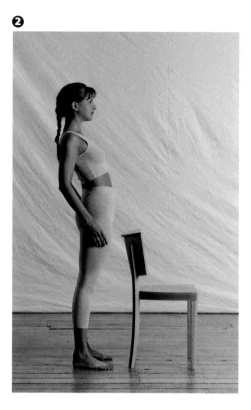

Shoulder shrug

Standing with your feet hips' width apart, your knees slightly bent, and your arms hanging by your side, lift up your chest a little and shake your shoulders and arms (1). Imagine that you are cold and your shoulders and arms are shivering. After doing this for 10 to 15 seconds, do slow, gentle shoulder shrugs, moving your shoulders backward. Lift your shoulders up toward your ears, and keep your shoulders high as you roll them backward (2), then relax your shoulders so that your hands drop further down toward your knees. Repeat this exercise six times.

Wall push

Stand facing the wall, with your feet about one foot (30 cm) away and balanced under your hips. Lift up your chest a little, tightening your buttocks. Bend your elbows and reach forward with your arms so your forearms rest against the wall – they should be parallel and shoulders' width apart (1).

Push into the wall with your forearms and maintain this pressure as you slowly slide your forearms up the wall about five inches (13 cm) (2). Keep your chest lifted as you slowly slide your arms back down the wall. Make sure you don't shrug your shoulders up toward your ears. Repeat this exercise six times.

This exercise works the muscles around your shoulder blades, and sometimes you may even feel a slight burn in this area.

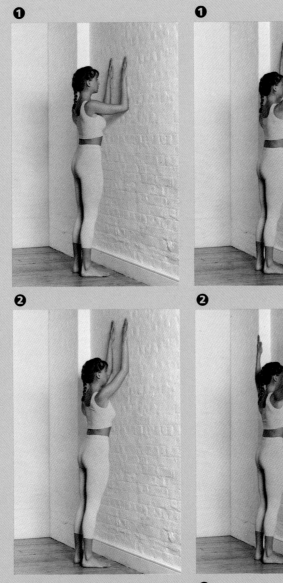

Wall push and drop

Stand facing the wall, with your feet about one foot (30 cm) away and balanced under your hips. Lift your chest a little and tighten your buttocks. Bend your elbows and reach forward with your arms so your forearms are resting against the wall, with your forearms wider than shoulders' width apart.

Slowly slide your forearms up the wall for five inches (13 cm), maintaining the pressure (1). Once you have reached this position, move your forearms a little way back from the wall (2), keeping your chest lifted high, your shoulder blades tucked down, and your elbows up. Now, slowly lower your arms back down (3). Repeat this exercise 10 times.

A slight burning feeling around the shoulder blades is normal and means you are working the correct muscles, but you should not feel pain.

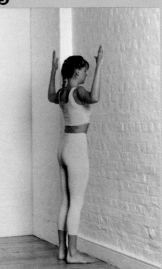

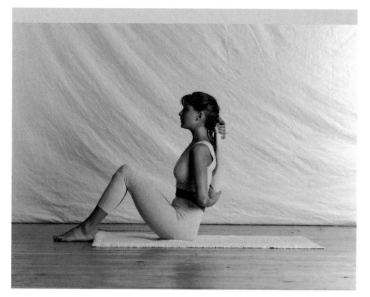

Towel stretch

Lie on your back (with your head resting on a pillow if you want), your knees bent, and your feet flat on the floor. Place a rolled towel beneath you along your spine, from the base of your neck to just below the bottom of your shoulder blades. You should feel balanced on the towel and not twisted to either side.

In this position, do nothing – just breathe deeply and allow your shoulders to relax over the rolled towel. You may feel some stretch around your shoulders or at the front of your chest. This is a good sign and means that the joints are gradually becoming more supple, and the tight muscles are stretching. Remain in this position for up to 10 minutes.

Consider it a relaxing time. It is best to do this exercise at the end of the day, but do not do it in bed, because you need to be resting on a firm surface to achieve the most benefit.

Bath stretch

This exercise stretches the nerve tissue in your spinal cord as it connects down your leg. It also stretches the joints between your ribs and the vertebrae in your upper back.

Sitting on the floor, with your knees slightly bent and a pillow or a rolled towel beneath them, cross your arms across your chest. Allow yourself to slouch and in this slouched position, twist your body to the left. Hold this stretch for 10 seconds, then repeat to the right. Do this exercise three or four times to each side. When you are more supple, you can remove the pillow and sit with your knees straight and your legs stretched out in front. However, if you experience an uncomfortable stretch in the backs of your legs or tingling in your feet, then this stretch is not for you.

Body spin
Sitting in a chair with your feet flat on the floor, your arms raised to shoulder level with your hands meeting in front of you, turn your head to the left, then follow with your shoulders. Stretch around as far as you can, as if you were straining to see something behind you. Hold this stretch for 10 seconds, then repeat on the opposite side. Do a total of three twists to each side.

Lower back strength

The muscles of your lower back play a crucial role in stabilizing the lower part of the spine and the pelvis. If they are working well, there will be very little strain to the joints and disks of your back, but when they are not, you will experience increased strain on your lower spine and, sooner or later, some back pain. This is because the muscles act to hold your spine up against gravity. They also work as shock absorbers, taking the body's weight as you walk or run.

These exercises must be repeated a minimum of 15 times each. Do the exercises slowly and think about the position of your lower back in relation to your pelvis and upper back. Try to visualize these muscles getting stronger as you do each repetition.

You should not feel any extra back pain either during the exercises or immediately after finishing them. With continued practice, you will note your posture improving and any back pain disappearing.

❶

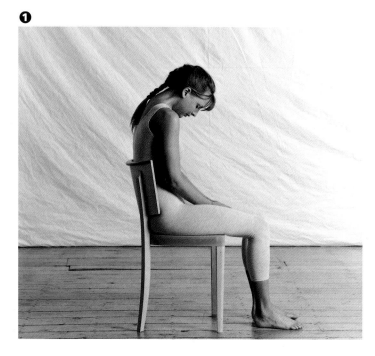

❷

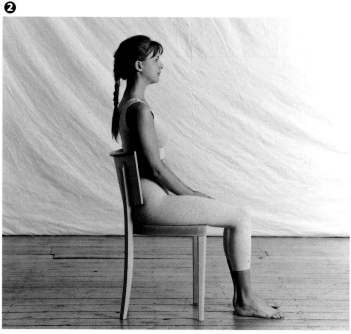

The extender
This is a great exercise to do whenever you are sitting down, and is also a warm-up for the other back strengthening exercises.
   Sitting on a chair with a slouched posture, keep your feet flat on the floor (1). By squeezing your buttocks, you will feel that you are rising a little in your chair. Continuing to squeeze your buttocks, lift your chest, straightening up from the slouched position and feeling even taller, using your lower back muscles to raise your body (2). Hold for 20 seconds, then relax and repeat.

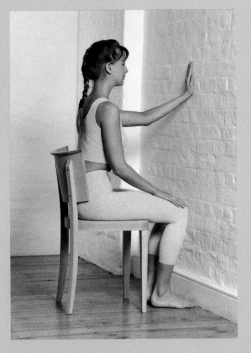

Strength push

Sit in a chair facing a wall, with your buttocks squeezed and your chest lifted, breathing easily from your lower chest. With your left arm, push your hand into the wall as if you were trying to push the wall away, but do not let any movement occur in your trunk or spine. The muscles of your lower back will be resisting the twisting movement that you are attempting by pushing the wall away. Hold this contraction for 15 seconds and then repeat with your right arm. Repeat four times on each side.

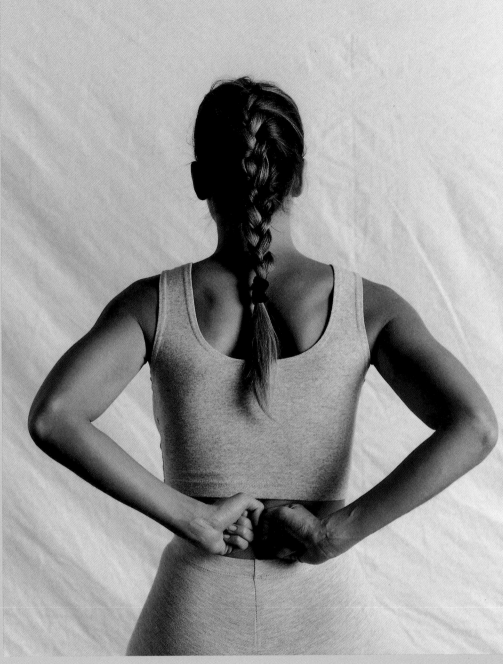

The back pump

Sitting in a tall position with your buttocks squeezed and your chest lifted, and breathing easily from your lower chest, rest your knuckles just on either side of your spine. Tighten your abdominal muscles, but don't hold your breath. As you do this, you should feel your muscles swelling underneath your thumbs. If you have a particular area of lower back pain, place your knuckles there; if you don't, move your knuckles up and down, working at different levels. Hold the muscle swell for 15 seconds, and repeat four or five times.

Lower back stretch

Most people will experience some stiffness in their lower back at some time, either with or without pain. This stiffness occurs when the muscles of the lower back are not working efficiently, causing strain. To avoid this, it is important to stretch out the muscles and joints of the lower back at the same time as you do strengthening exercises.

You should choose only three or four of these exercises to incorporate into your daily routine. It is good to feel a stretch in your lower back when you are performing these exercises, but if you feel any pain or discomfort, you should not push the exercise any further: just relax and breathe deeply, and the discomfort should pass.

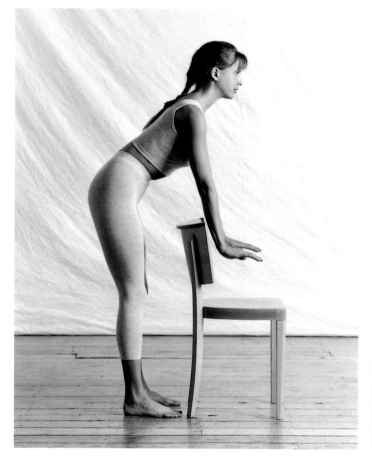

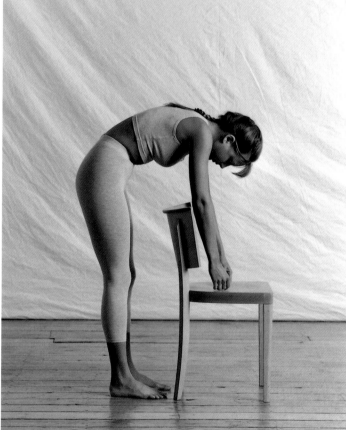

Waiter's bow
Stand behind a chair with your weight equally on both feet and your feet aligned under your hips. Squeeze your buttocks and hollow your lower abdominal muscles by contracting them before you begin any movement. Keeping your back straight, lean forward from the hips, slowly sliding your hands down the back of the chair and letting the chair guide your movement. When you have gone as low as you can, hold the stretch for 10 seconds before slowly returning to the standing position, keeping your back straight.

Puppet
Imagine yourself suspended by strings like a puppet. Think how it would feel if the strings supporting the top of your body broke.
   Stand behind the back of the chair with your weight equally on both feet. Starting with your head, curl forward so your chin touches your chest, then continue the curling movement from your upper back down, slowly curling until you have gone as far as you can. At this point hold the stretch for 10 seconds. On the way back up, gently uncurl from your lower back to your upper back, then your neck and finally your head.

Chair twist

Stand facing a chair and place your left foot on the seat. Slowly bend forward, reaching inside your bent knee as you come forward. You will feel yourself twisting toward the right from your hips. Don't bounce as you do this exercise – slowly and smoothly allow your body to go as far as it can naturally. Repeat this exercise six times on each side.

Sciatic back stretch

This exercise will stretch the sciatic nerve, which runs from the base of your head to the back of your leg and foot. You should not experience tingling in your leg or pain in your back when you do this exercise.

Sit on a chair and slouch, allowing your chin to tuck onto your chest. Slowly straighten your left leg, flexing your foot. Stop as soon as you feel a gentle pull in the back of your leg. Hold this position for three seconds, then place your left foot back on the floor before returning to a tall sitting position. Repeat on the opposite leg. Do no more than two repetitions on each leg.

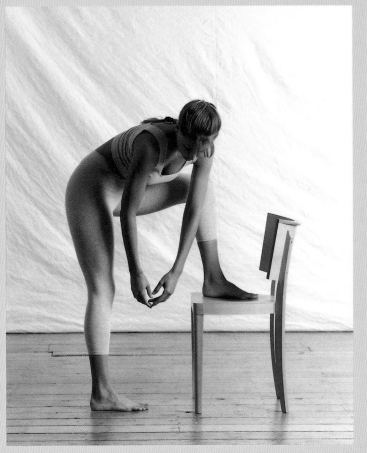

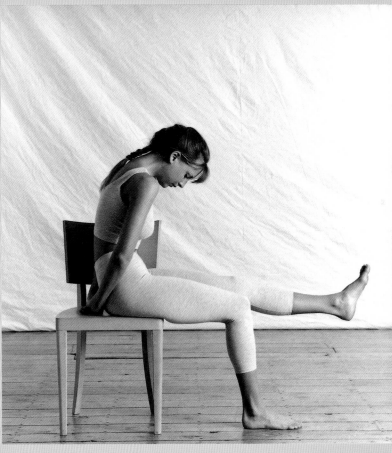

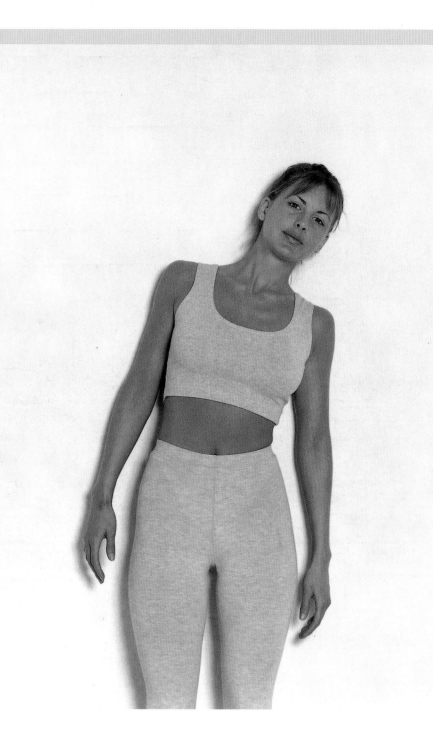

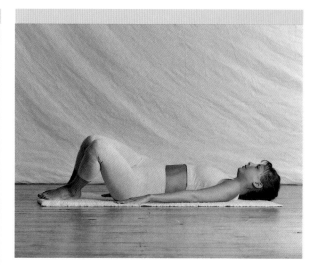

Back roll

Lie flat on your back with both knees bent, feet flat on the floor, and your arms by your sides. Slowly allow both of your legs to fall toward the left, stretching the right side of your back, until your left leg rests on the floor. Stop if you feel any discomfort in your lower back. Hold this position for six seconds, and repeat three times on each side.

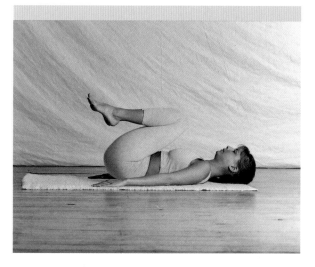

Double hip curl

Lying flat on your back, bring both your knees toward your chest and clasp them with your hands. Pull gently on your legs to help curl your knees up toward your chest. You should have rolled up into a ball. Hold this position for 20 seconds before relaxing to the floor. Repeat three times.

Wall slide

Stand with your back to a wall, leaning against it, with your feet two foot-lengths away and your knees slightly bent. Tighten your low abdominal muscles and flatten your lower back against the wall, imagining a brace holding your lower back flat against the wall. Slowly allow your left hand to reach down toward your left knee, bending your upper body to the side as you go. Reach as low as you can, holding the stretch for 10 seconds, before slowly sliding back to the starting position. Repeat six times on each side.

Hip curl

Lying flat on your back, bend your right leg up toward your chest, and reach down with your hands to clasp your knee. Lightly pull your knee in toward your chest, feeling a gentle stretch in the small of your back and right buttock. Hold this position for 20 seconds, before relaxing to the floor. Repeat three times on each leg.

Cobra

Lie face down on the floor with your weight through your forearms, elbows bent and under your shoulders. Pushing through your forearms, lift your head and chest high, and the small of your back will arch gently. Hold for 30 seconds, then relax back to the floor before repeating three times.

For a more advanced version of this stretch, place your hands underneath your shoulders as you lie face-down. Slowly lift your head and shoulders and then push through your hands to straighten your elbows (see picture). Your upper back should arch first, followed by your lower back. Keep the front of your hips on the floor. Stop as soon as you feel a stretch in your lower back, or if you cannot arch any further because of stiffness. Hold this position for 30 seconds and repeat three times. If you experience any lower back pain during this exercise, return to the basic stretch until you are more supple.

Abdominals

The abdominal muscles are essential in supporting the trunk. By strengthening them, you lessen your chances of lower back strain, because the abs and the lower back work in partnership.

Because the abs are a group of four different muscles, you have to do a variety of different kinds of exercises if you want to work them all. For example, twisting movements work the obliques at the side of the trunk, while crunches act on the muscles to the front of the abdomen.

With all these exercises, it is important to work slowly and carefully. Do not move to the more advanced exercises until you are strong and confident, and if you feel any lower back pain during one of the exercises, stop immediately and spend a few more sessions working on easier variations before trying that exercise again.

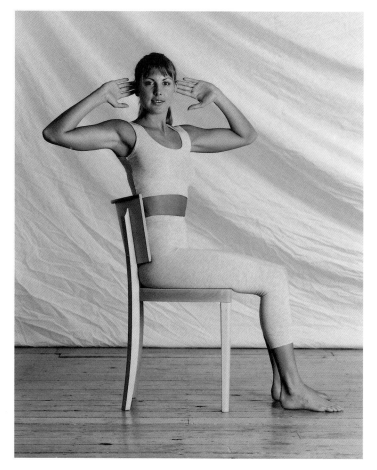

Seated twist
Sit on a firm chair, your feet flat on the floor, and rest your hands near your ears with your elbows pointing out. Twist so your left arm and elbow come across your body, without bending forward or tilting. You should feel your abdominals working, as well as a slight stretch in your upper back. Hold for a few seconds, before relaxing and repeating on the other side.

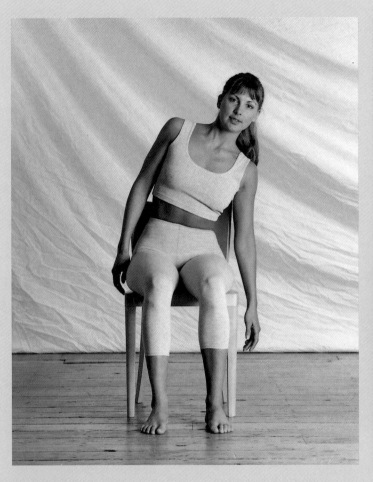

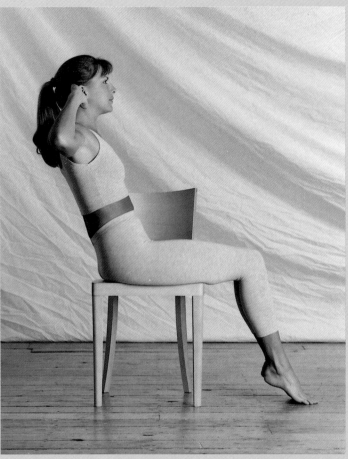

Side bend

Sit toward the edge of the seat of a firm chair, your feet flat on the floor and your arms relaxed by your side. Without tilting forward, bend to the left, lowering your left hand toward the floor. Straighten up before lowering your body to the right. Repeat 10 times on each side.

See saw

Sit on a firm chair, with your hands behind your head, elbows out to the side, and your feet flat on the floor. Keep your back straight as you slowly tilt forward from the waist, then straighten up before tilting backward. Repeat 10 to 12 times, continuing to move slowly and evenly. If you have any lower back pain, stop and relax, and come back to.this exercise a few weeks later.

Chair march
Sitting on a firm chair with your feet flat on the floor, lean backward, keeping your back straight. Slowly raise one leg, keeping your foot and knee in line with your hip, and lower it before repeating with the other leg. Repeat 10 times on each leg. To make this exercise more challenging, you can lean back further or lift your leg higher.

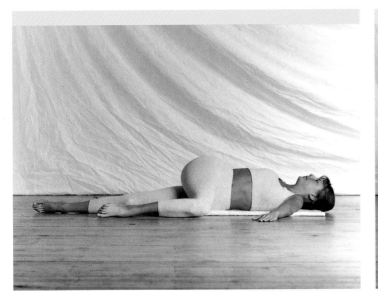

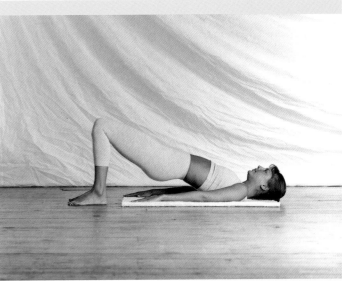

Lying leg roll

This is a good stretch for the lower back and back of the thighs. Lie on your back, with both legs straight, and your arms gently stretched out at shoulder level and resting on the floor, so your body makes a "T" shape. Bend your right knee and and lift your right leg up and over your body to roll toward the left. Hold this position for six seconds, before relaxing and repeating three times on each side.

Abdominal tilt

Lie on your back on the floor with your knees bent and your feet, knees, and hips in line with each other. Keeping your feet and shoulders still and squeezing your buttocks, raise your pelvis and lower back into the air in one slow, controlled motion, until the front of your body, from your thighs through your abs and chest, makes a flat plane, then lower yourself back slowly to the ground. Repeat 10 times.

Basic crunch

Lying on your back with your knees bent and your feet flat on the floor, and your hands resting by your ears, tighten your lower abdominal muscles and, keeping your lower back stable and on the floor, curl up slowly, head and upper back first, until you reach the limit of your movement. Don't lead from your head – make sure you keep your neck aligned with your spine, working from your abdominals. Relax down to the floor, then repeat 10 times in total.

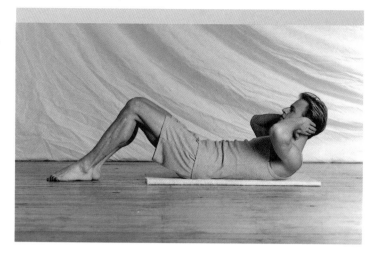

Side lying oblique

This exercise works your obliques on the side of your trunk. It will help to trim your waist and give more support to your spine. Begin by lying on your left side with your knees bent and in line with your hips, then turn your upper body so your head and shoulders are flat on the floor, and rest your hands by your ears. Crunch up, moving first from the head then your upper chest, middle chest, and finally your lower back, then relax down, reversing the process, moving slowly and smoothly throughout. Repeat 10 times on each side.

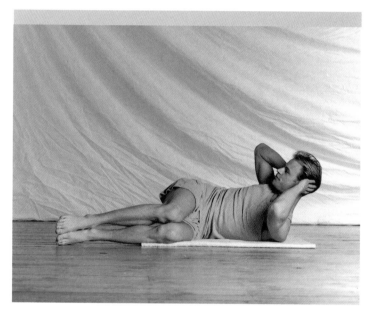

Side bending toe reach

Lying on your back with your knees bent and feet flat, lift your head and shoulders slowly off the floor and bend down and sideways so your left hand reaches toward your left foot. Return to the center, keeping your head and shoulders off the floor, then bend toward the right side. Don't try to stretch too far – it is only a small movement. Repeat 10 times on each side.

High toe reach

This is an advanced exercise, which you should only try once you have mastered the other abs exercises.

Lie on your back with your feet pointing toward the ceiling, with your ankles crossed, your knees relaxed and slightly bent, and your left arm under your head. Slowly lift your head and shoulders from the floor and reach to your feet with your right hand. Return to the floor before repeating on the other side. Repeat as many times as you can on each side.

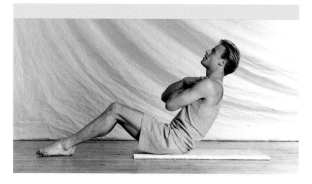

Body lowering

Sit on the floor with your knees slightly bent and pointing up to the ceiling, and cross your hands on your chest. Slowly lower your upper body to the floor for a count of 10, keeping your back straight. Try to keep the movement slow and even. As you become stronger you will be able to take 15 or even 20 seconds to lower your upper body to the ground.

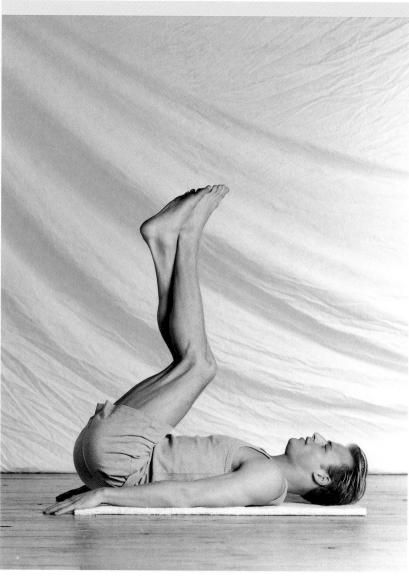

Reverse curl

Lying on your back with knees bent, ankles crossed, and feet flat, tighten your low abdominal muscles and, keeping your back in a natural position, neither arched nor flattened, breathe in and bring your knees slowly up toward your chest. Hold for a few seconds then slowly uncurl as you breathe out, until your feet rest on the floor.

You may do this exercise up to 15 times. The aim is to work on your lower stomach muscles.

❶

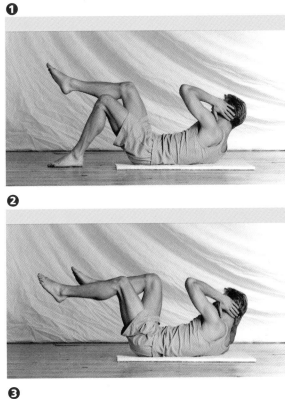

❷

❸

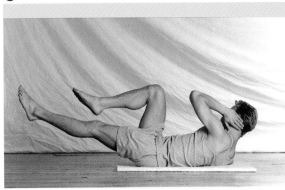

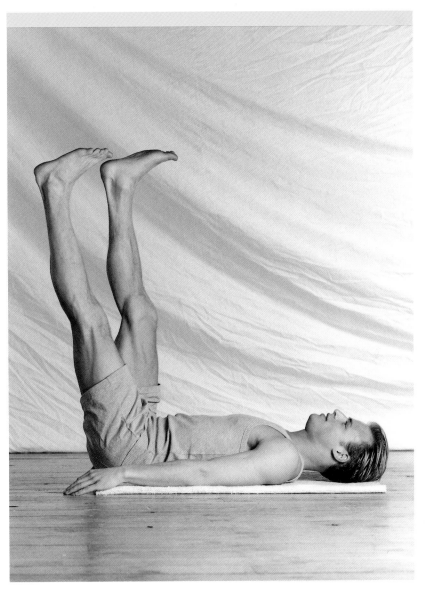

Sprinter

This is an advanced exercise, and you should be very careful to move slowly, smoothly, and with control.

Lying on your back with your knees bent and your hands resting by your ears, lift your right leg so your thigh is vertical. Moving up into the crunch position, twist your upper body so your left elbow moves toward your right knee, and at the same time move your right knee toward your left elbow (1). Relax to the floor, before switching sides. When you are strong enough, you can do the same movement, keeping both legs off the floor (2), or try extending the left leg as you reach toward the right knee with the left elbow (3). Remember to do the same number of repetitions on both sides.

Back walk

Lie on your back on the floor, with your legs straight up in the air and feet flexed. Move your legs back and forth from the hips, as if you were taking very small steps, keeping your feet flexed. Continue for 30 seconds, then bend your knees before lowering your legs back on the floor and relaxing.

Warm-ups

Before you play any sport or begin any general exercise routine, such as a game of tennis, a run, or exercise from a video, it is important to warm up. This will prepare you for more vigorous activity, because the muscles will be supple and active and the joints will be more flexible.

These exercises will prepare the muscles of your lower back and stomach to support you easily during your exercise and will increase the flexibility of your lower back. They are particularly useful for those who are returning to sport after experiencing back pain.

You do not need to do the entire warm-up before your sporting activity: just spend around five minutes and choose five or six exercises.

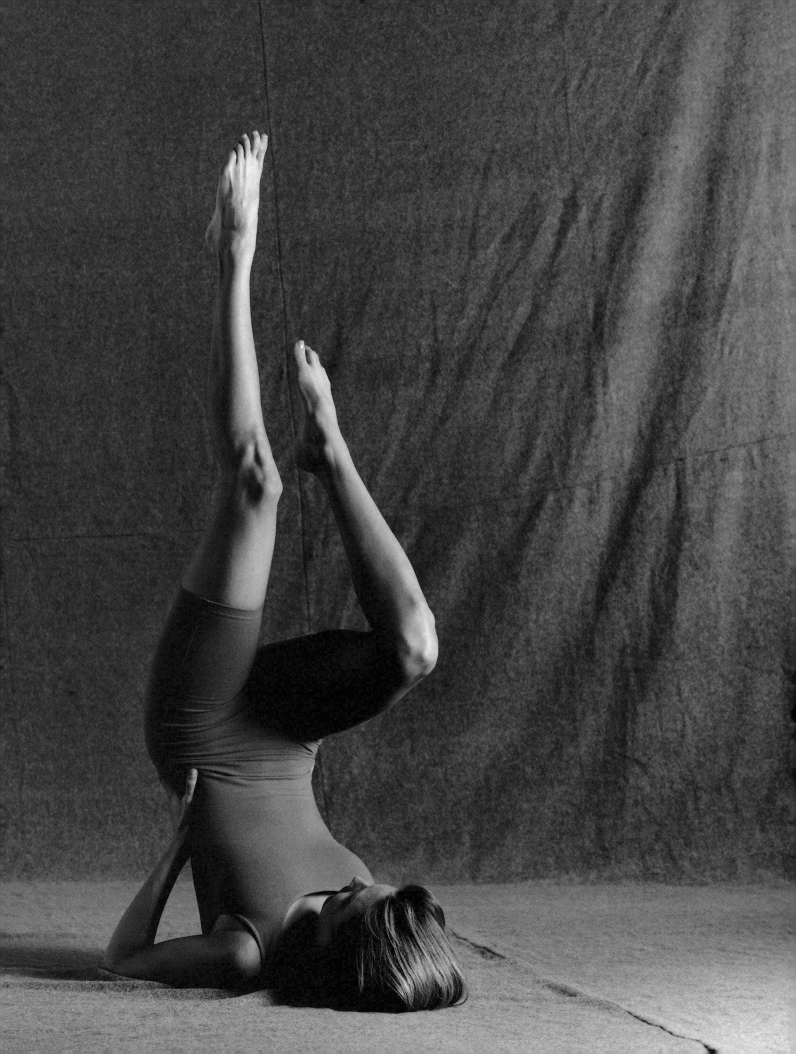

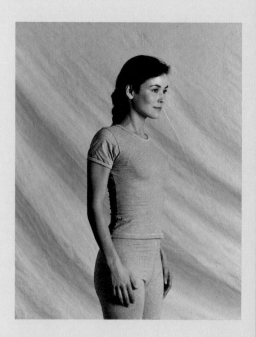

Shoulder shrug
Standing with your weight equally divided over both legs, shrug your shoulders up toward your ears, then roll your shoulders backward, without lifting your arms. Repeat these small circles six times, keeping your head still and centered.

Windmill
Standing with your weight divided equally over both legs, swing both your arms to the front of your body, keeping your elbows straight. Continue the arm swing so your arms move up over your head and then back behind your body. Repeat this movement five or six times, making the circles progressively larger, faster, and more fluid.

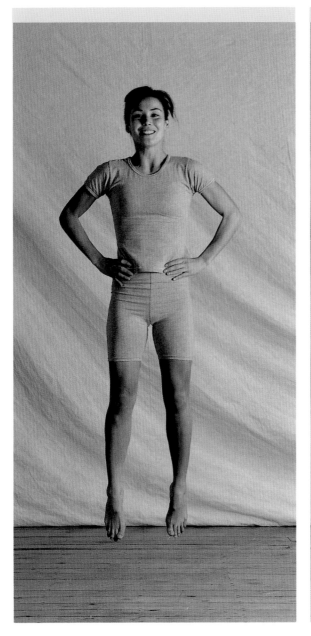

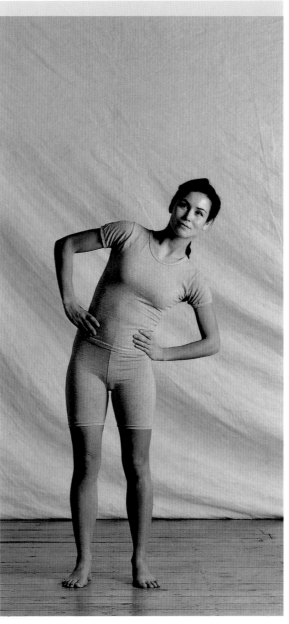

Basketballer

Standing with your weight divided equally over both legs, bend slightly at your hips and knees, then straighten your legs again so that you stand up tall. Repeat this movement 15 times. You should feel the muscles on your thighs working, but there should not be any knee pain. When you feel loose and comfortable, begin to make little jumps as you straighten your knees.

Military warm-up

Stand tall, with your feet hips' width apart and your hands on your hips. Keeping your body stable, bend slowly to the left so you feel a stretch on the right side of your torso. Return to the center and repeat on the right side. Repeat six times in total, alternating left and right sides.

❶

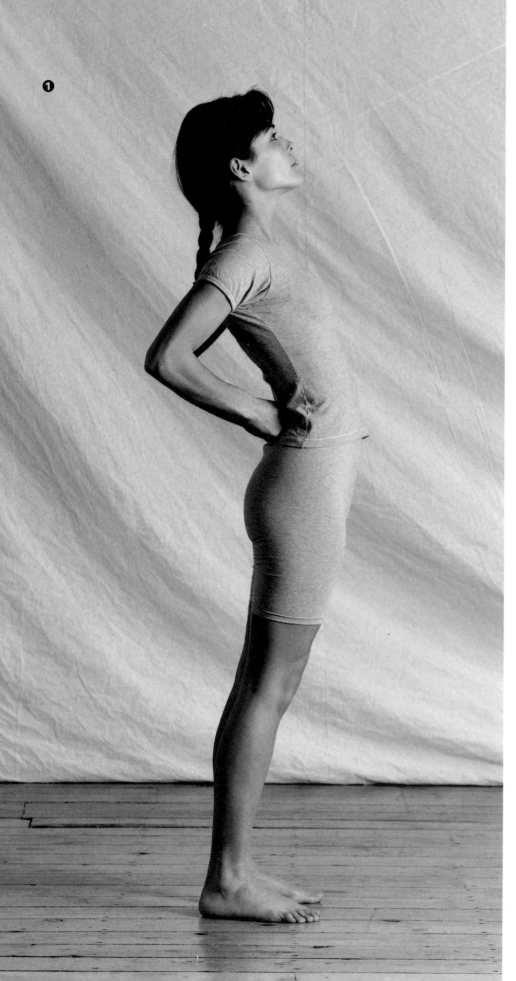

❷

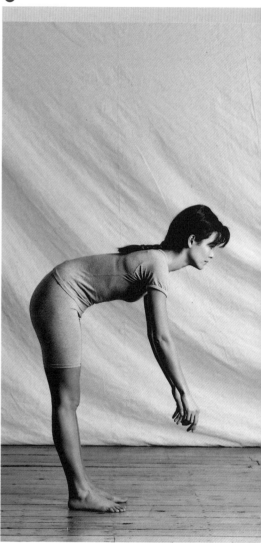

Cobra bow

Standing with feet hips' width apart, resting your fists in the small of your back, arch backward (1). Keep your head facing to the front, so you do not throw it backward. Straighten up, then curl forward from the waist, letting your arms fall freely (2). Do not push this stretch too far – your back and thighs should feel comfortable throughout. Return to standing and relax. Repeat six times.

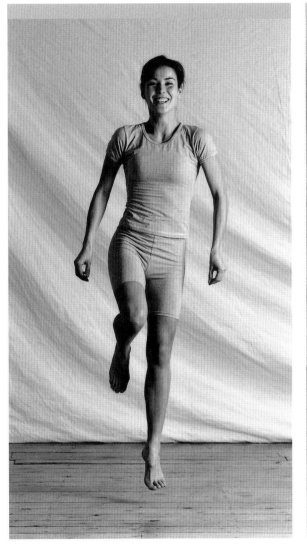

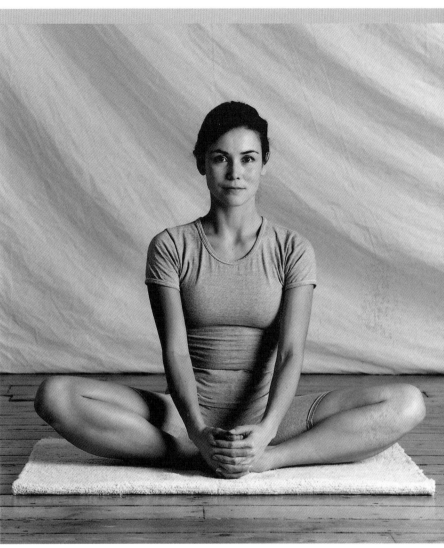

Grasshopper

This simple exercise works the lower back, buttocks, calf, and thigh muscles. Balancing on your right leg, gently hop, allowing your hip and knee to bend through a comfortable range. Hop 10 times on one leg, then 10 times on the other leg.

Butterfly

Sit on the floor, knees bent, so the soles of your feet rest against each other. Reach down with your hands and hold your ankles or your feet. Sit tall, allowing your knees to fall out. You should feel a stretch in your inner thighs and low back. Hold this position for 15 seconds, before relaxing and repeating three times.

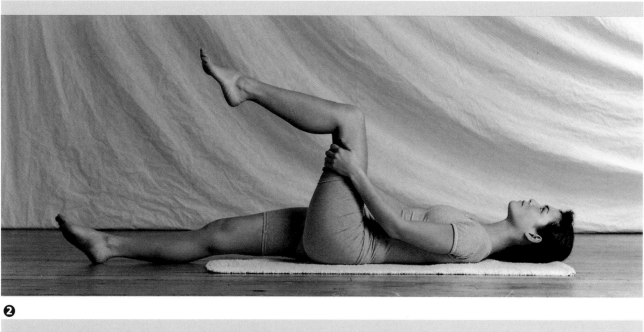

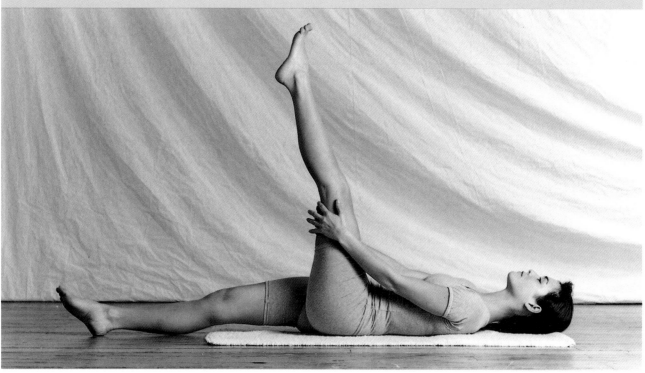

Hamstring stretch

This exercise stretches the muscles at the back of your thigh.
Lying on your back, reach down to clasp your left leg, behind the
knee (1). Bend at your hip so your thigh is vertical, and slowly
straighten your left knee, without straining (2). Allow your foot
to relax, and hold the stretch for 15 seconds. Repeat three times
on each leg.

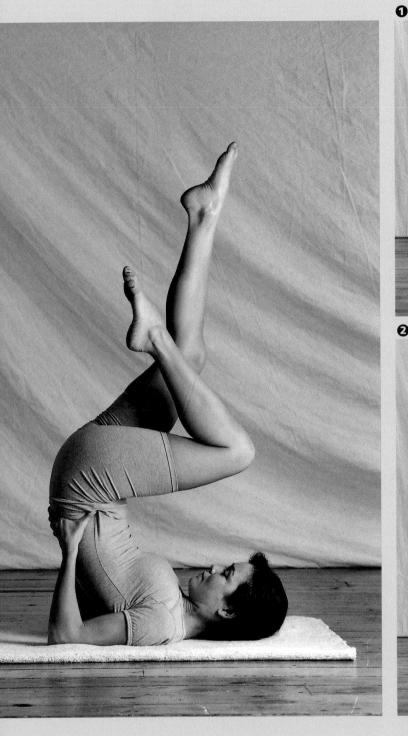

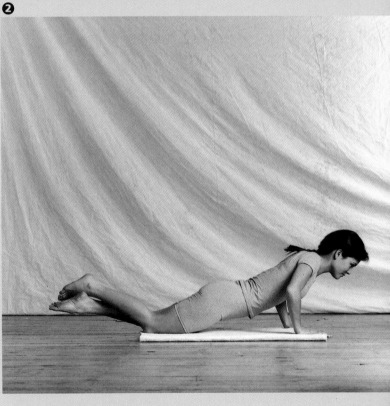

Bicycle

This is good preparation for any running activities. Lying on your back, lift your legs up, bracing yourself by placing your hands in the small of your back and resting on your elbows. In this position your legs should be above your chest. Make slow circles with your legs, as if you were riding a bicycle upside down. Continue for 20 seconds, have a rest, and repeat this exercise twice. You will find this works your low abdominal and back muscles, as well as your thigh muscles.

Easy push-up

This exercise works your upper back and chest muscles as well as your buttock muscles. Lying face down on the floor, with your hands under your shoulders, take your weight on your hands and your knees, balancing between them and keeping your back straight (1). Push up through your arms, moving your chest away from the floor, then lower your body back to the floor by bending your elbows (2). Repeat 10 times.

Prayer

Kneel on the floor with your weight divided equally over your hands and knees. Shift your body back, keeping your hands flat on the floor, and curling your chin down onto your chest. Hold the stretch for 10 seconds before returning to the starting position and repeating three times.

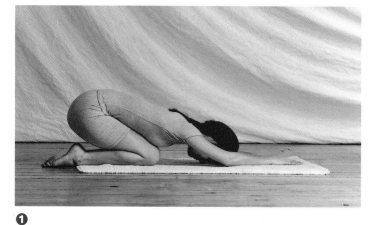

Advanced crawl

Resting on your hands and knees, keep your back stable and your weight balanced over both of your hands and left knee as you bend your right knee up toward your chest and tuck your chin down, curling your back (1). Then, extend your right leg out behind you and lift your head, making sure your back remains straight and strong (2). Repeat six times with the right leg, then six times with the left. This will improve the suppleness of your whole spine.

❶

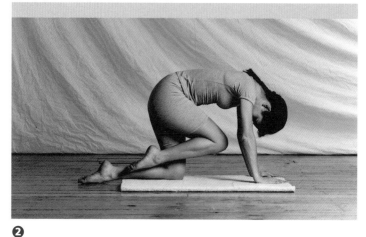

❷

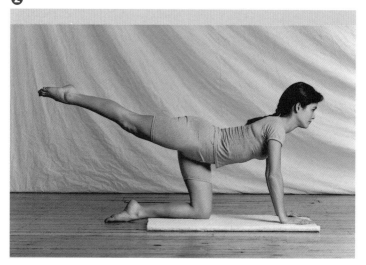

Star jumps

This is a good exercise to do toward the end of your sporting warm-up. It will increase your heart rate, improve the blood flow to your arms and legs, and make the muscles in your back, buttocks, and thighs work to support your spine.

Standing with your weight equally divided over both legs, jump up in the air at the same time as you open your legs and throw both your arms up above your head. You may clap your hands above your head as you do this.

Land on the floor with feet still apart and hands above your head, then jump up into the air again, bringing your feet together and your arms back down by your sides, before landing again.

Repeat for a few minutes. You may increase the speed of the exercise as you get stronger and fitter.

Total body workout

For your body to move efficiently, it must have a strong and stable base for the limbs. When a runner gets tired, the trunk and pelvis muscles fatigue first, putting more stress on the back and legs. Similarly, an office worker who sits at a desk all day will also find that trunk and pelvis muscles weaken. This may cause stress on the spine and on the nerves from the neck to the arms, resulting in neck pain and headache.

These exercises increase the stability of your trunk and pelvis by working the muscles of the lower back, the stomach, and the buttocks. You will develop greater awareness of how your trunk and pelvis move and relate to the movements of your arms and legs.

Each day, take a few minutes to do three or four exercises from the torso group and one or two from the buttocks and pelvis and abdominal groups.

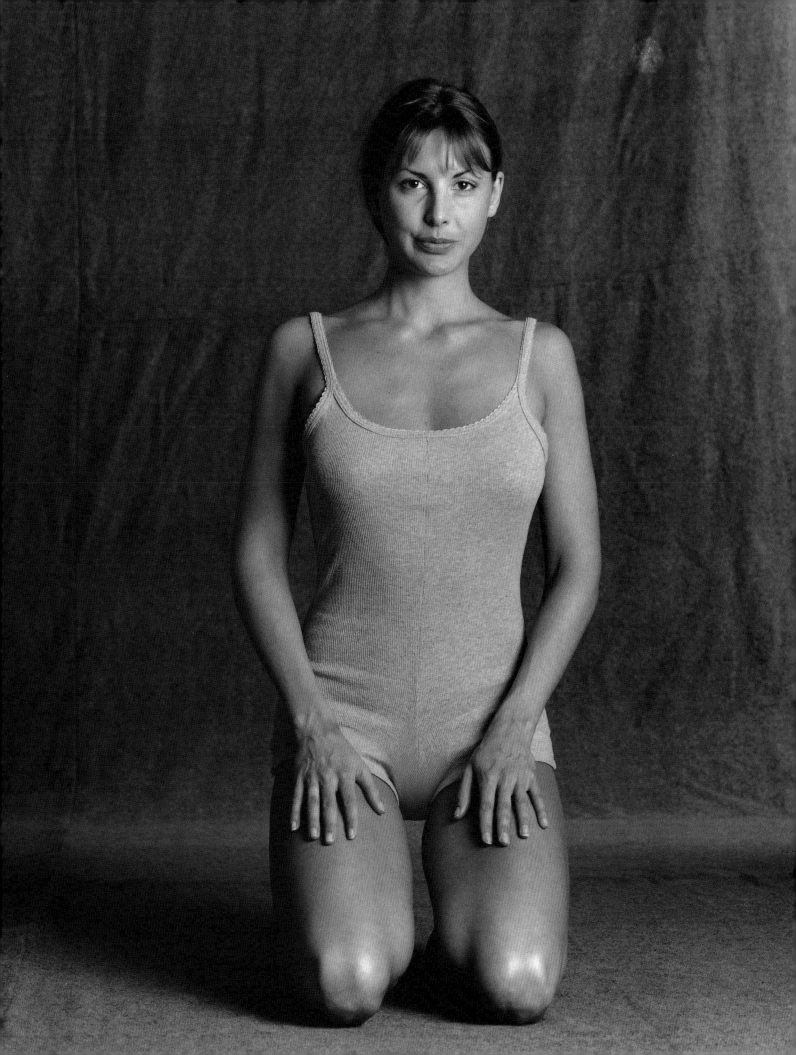

Torso

Your torso – your abdominals, back, chest, and shoulders – is the basis around which your limbs move and is your center of gravity and balance. Therefore, in order to move effectively and efficiently, you must develop the strength and the stability of your torso. The exercises in this section help to enhance the strength and flexibility of the different muscle groups in your trunk, and to improve ways in which these various muscles work intricately together.

❶

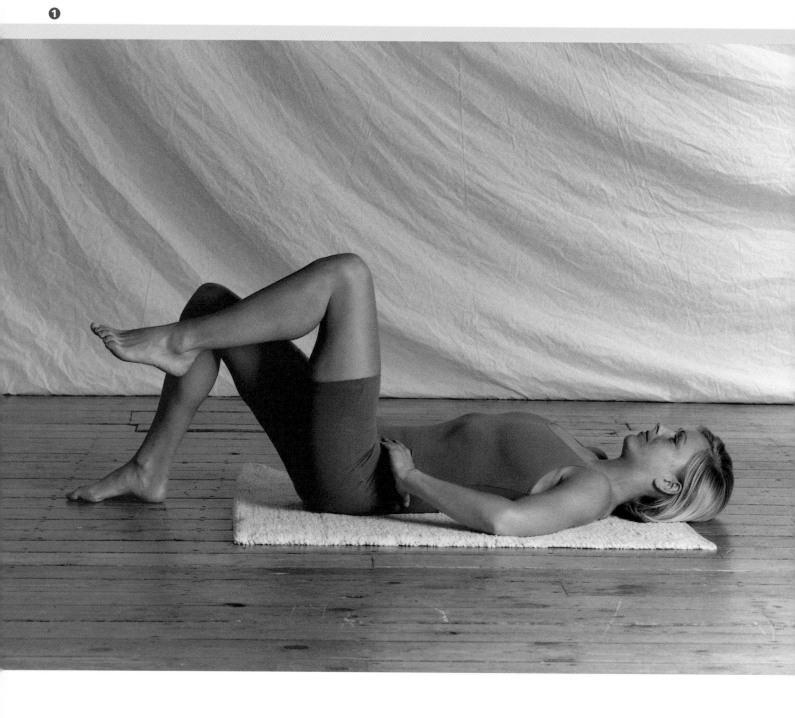

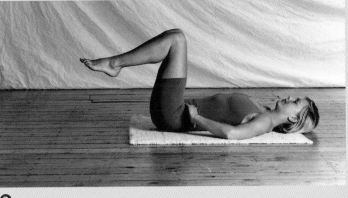

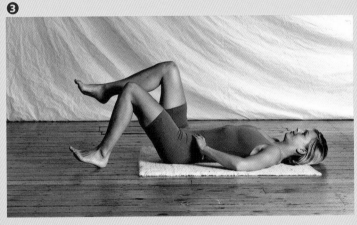

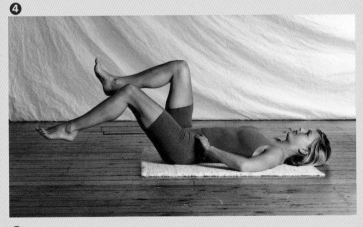

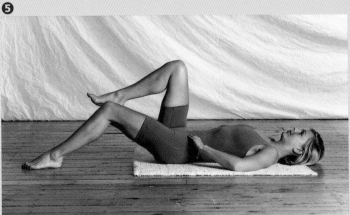

Lying knee lifts

Lie flat on your back with knees bent, your feet and knees in line with your hips, and your feet flat on the floor. It is important that you keep your back straight when you do this, and that there is no movement in your upper body.

1. Lift up your left leg, so your knee is above your hip. Hold this position for 10 seconds, then slowly lower your left leg to the starting position, before switching to the right leg. Repeat this 10 times on each leg. This exercise works the hip flexors and low abdominal muscles.

2. Lift your left leg so your knee is above your hip, and keep your left leg in this position as you lift your right leg to join it.

3. Keeping both your legs in this position and your trunk stable, lower your left leg slowly until your heel touches the floor. Raise your left leg before repeating with the right leg. Repeat 10 times on each leg. This exercise works to strengthen your low abdominal muscles and lower back muscles.

4. This variation should only be done by people with no back pain and who play sport at some level – gymnasts do this exercise regularly. Starting with both your knees above your hips and your back straight and stable, lower your left leg first, but don't let it touch the ground. Keep it slightly off the ground as you slide it out, again making sure that your foot, knee, and hips stay in line and your back remains still. Repeat this exercise six times only on each leg. If you experience any back pain at all, stop right away.

5. Starting with both your knees above your hips and your back stable, slowly lower your left leg so your left foot touches the floor, and, keeping your left foot in contact with the floor, allow your leg to slide down until it is not quite straight. Keep your foot, knee, and hip in line, and do not allow your leg to roll inward. Slowly slide your foot back toward your body and lift your foot so your knee is again above your hip. Repeat on the right leg. Do this exercise 10 times on each side.

❶

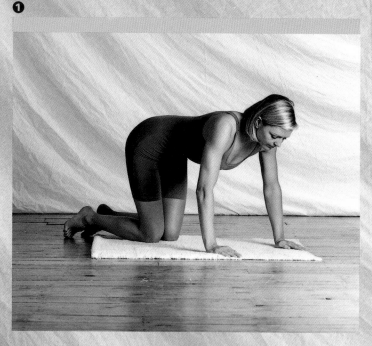

The crawler

Kneel on your hands and knees with your hands under your shoulders, your knees in line with your hips, and your spine straight. The movement is subtle: you should push through your arms to keep your chest raised from the floor (1). Make sure your head is facing forward and not flopped down toward the floor. Hold this position for 15 seconds, and repeat five times.

This exercise works the muscles around your shoulder blades that help to keep your shoulders and neck in a good position. You should not feel any neck or arm pain while you are doing this. If you do, try to work a little more gently, but make sure you stop if the pain persists.

As an advanced variation, you can move your body weight in a diagonal so your weight presses more over the your left hand and your right knee (2). Hold this position for six seconds, then repeat on the other diagonal. Do this exercise at least six times on each side. If you are right-handed, then you should focus on doing two or three more exercises to the right side, and if you are left-handed, you should work a little more to the left.

❷

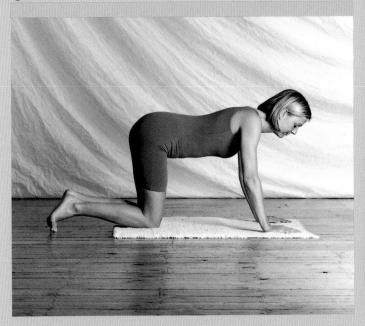

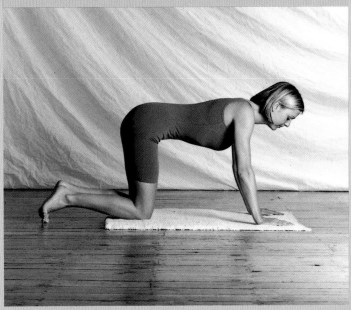

Tummy tuck

Begin on your hands and knees, with your hands in line with your shoulders, your knees in line with your hips, and your spine straight. Keep your head facing forward.

Allow your abdominals to relax so your belly flops down toward the floor (1). Keeping your spine stable, breathe in, allowing your breath to reach all the way down to your stomach. As you breathe out, squeeze your pelvic floor muscles and hollow your low abdominal muscles (2). Do not suck in your whole stomach – the only part of your stomach that should move is the very low part next to your pelvis. As you hold your low stomach hollowed, keep breathing easily. Hold for 20 seconds, relax, and repeat 10 to 12 times.

Bent knee fall-out

Lie on your back, with your hands resting lightly on your hipbones, your knees bent, and your feet flat on the floor. As you breathe out, let your left leg gently fall away from your body, but make sure your hips remain still – your hands will feel any movement. Hold for a few seconds, before breathing in and returning your leg to the starting position. Repeat 10 times on each leg.

Buttocks and pelvis

The buttock muscles coordinate the movement of your trunk, and your hips and legs. Parts of the buttock muscles are responsible for twisting the hip and leg outward, and others are responsible for moving your hip and leg backward. The muscles of your low abdomen work with the buttock muscles to stabilize the hips and trunk. These exercises will improve the stability of your pelvic region, strengthen the buttocks, and improve their appearance, and will increase mobility in your hips.

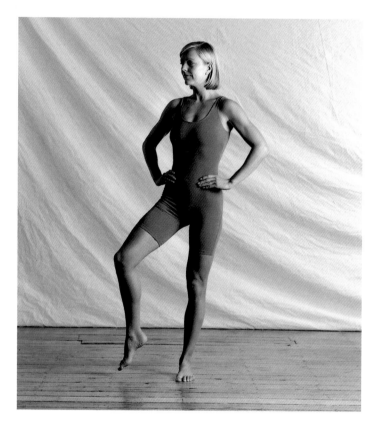

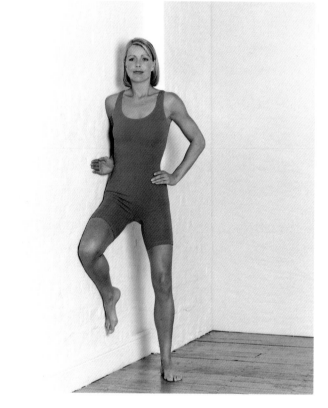

Turnaway

This exercise is slightly more difficult than the side buttock lift (opposite), which uses the same muscles, since it requires additional balance and coordination – but because you work against the force of gravity, it is more dynamic.

Stand with your weight on your left leg, with the knee slightly bent. Lift your right leg off the floor, and keeping your kneecap and foot facing straight ahead, turn your body to the right by pivoting on the left hip. Squeeze your left buttock as you do this movement. Hold this position for 10 seconds before relaxing and repeating six times on each side.

Get it together

This exercise is still more complex and requires a fair degree of trunk and pelvis stability. Stand with your right side to the wall and your right leg bent at the hip and knee. Push the right leg against the wall, and take all of your weight on the left leg.

Bend slightly at the left knee and make sure that your pelvis is facing straight ahead. Squeeze your left buttock and twist out from the left knee and hip. Keep your trunk and pelvis still. Hold this position for 20 seconds, before relaxing and repeating three times on each side. If you feel a twist in your trunk and pelvis, or if you feel unbalanced doing this exercise, go back to the easier exercises in this section for two weeks more before trying again.

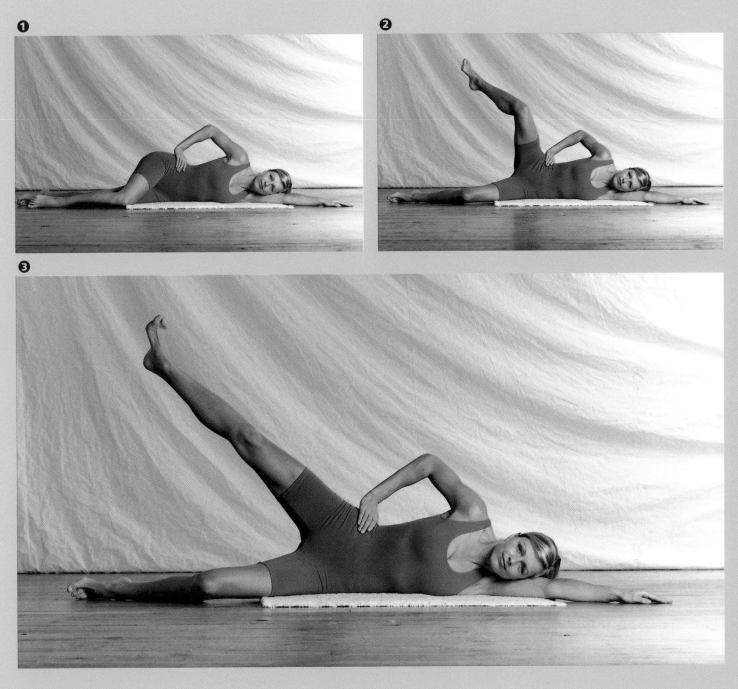

Side buttock lift

This exercise will work the muscles of your buttocks that are responsible for twisting your hip out.

Lying on your side with your bottom leg straight and top leg bent so your knee is almost level with your hip (1), tighten your low abdominal muscles, keeping your back straight. Slowly lift your top knee toward the ceiling, making sure your knee stays bent at the original angle and your trunk does not twist (2). Hold this position for six seconds, then relax. Repeat this exercise six times on each side.

You can vary this exercise by keeping your bottom knee bent and your top leg straight. As you lift your leg toward the ceiling, twist your foot out (3). Hold your leg up for six seconds before lowering it, relaxing, and repeating six times on each leg. Again, make sure your trunk does not twist.

Swimmer

Lying on your stomach with your head turned to one side, tighten your abdominals and your buttock muscles. Keeping both knees straight, raise one leg from the floor, lifting from the hip. Your foot should be no more than four inches (10 cm) from the floor. Do not compensate for the lift by pressing your upper body into the floor – all the movement should come from your hip and pelvis. Hold for 20 seconds before relaxing and repeating on the other leg.

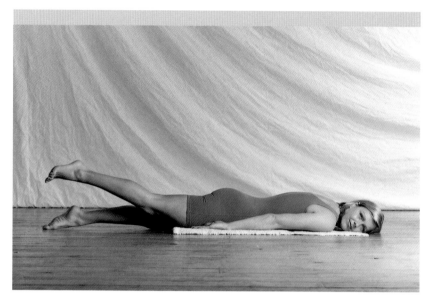

Hip hitch

Lying face down, bend your right knee so your foot is above your knee, gently hollow your low abdominal muscles, and squeeze your buttocks tight. Lift your right knee just one inch (2–3cm) off the floor, moving from your hip. Hold this position for 10 seconds before relaxing, and repeat 10 times on each side.

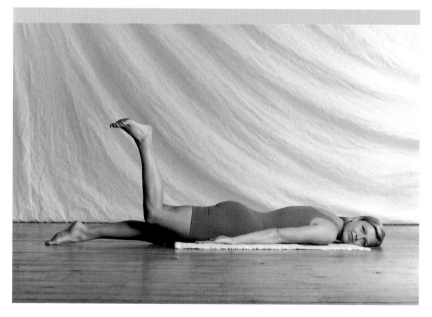

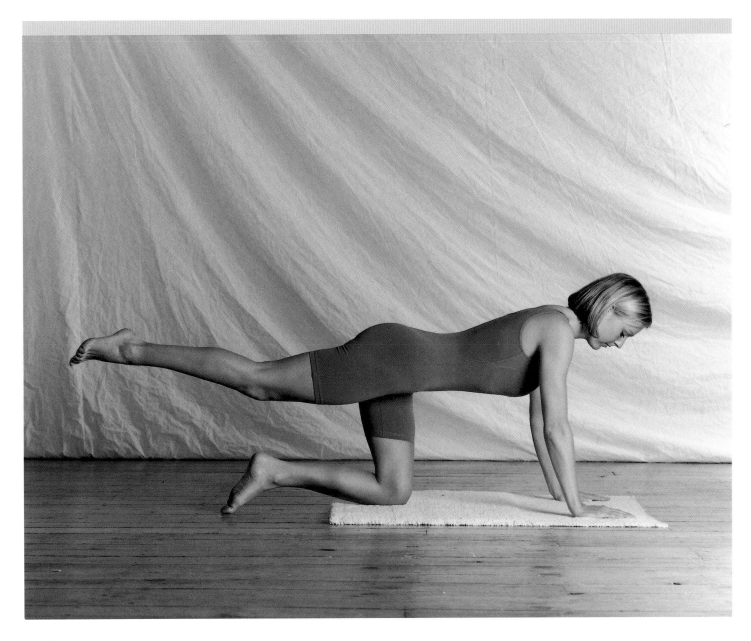

Kickback

This exercise works your abdominal and back muscles at the same time as it tones your buttock muscles.

On your hands and knees, tighten your lower abdominal muscles and keep your back straight and relaxed. Straighten your right knee and hip to raise your leg straight behind you as if kicking backward. Maintain this position for three seconds,

before relaxing and repeating six times on each leg. It is important to keep the rest of your body as stable as possible as you kick back with your moving leg.

As an advanced variation, you can reach up with your left arm at the same time as you reach back with your left leg. Again, hold for three seconds, and repeat six times on each leg.

Abdominals

The abdominals are the muscles running from the ribs down to the pelvis, and also from the spinal vertebrae of the lower back around to the front of the stomach. These muscles bend the trunk forward and maintain stability of the trunk in conjunction with the lower back muscles. If these muscles are flabby and weak, it is not only unattractive – you also risk suffering from lower back pain, because the muscles are not supporting your trunk. You should choose two or three exercises to do from this section. They are some of the most important exercises to include in your daily practice.

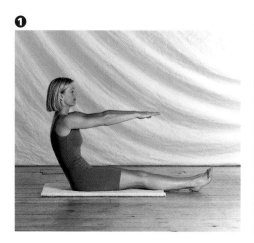

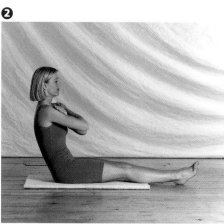

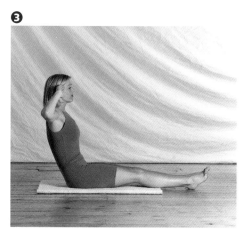

Toe reach

Lying flat on your back with your legs out straight, tighten your low abdominal muscles, and slowly curl up: drop your chin toward your chest, then curl from the top of your chest, reaching toward your toes (1). When you are sitting up, tighten your low abdominals again and slowly uncurl until you are lying flat. You can also vary the arm position to make the exercise more challenging, either crossing your arms across your chest (2), or placing your hands lightly against your temples (3).

Do not try this exercise if you get any lower back pain. At first, do not do too many repetitions. If your legs start to lift from the floor, it is a sure sign that you have done too much and your abdominals have fatigued. Breathe deeply to relax.

The crunch

Lying on your back with your hips and knees bent to right angles and your lower legs and feet resting on a sofa or chair, tighten your low abdominal muscles and keep your lower back stable. With arms folded across your chest or with your hands placed lightly against your temples, curl up slowly, head and upper back first, until you reach your limit. Hold this position for three seconds before slowly lowering your body to the floor.

Repeat this exercise with a slight twist, so that as you come up, your right shoulder moves toward your left knee. Next time, your left shoulder moves toward your right knee.

Repeat a maximum of 15 times, stopping if you get tired.

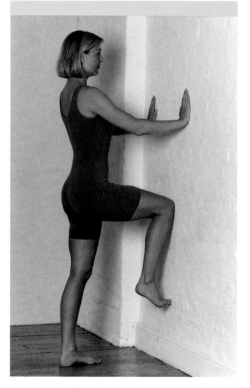

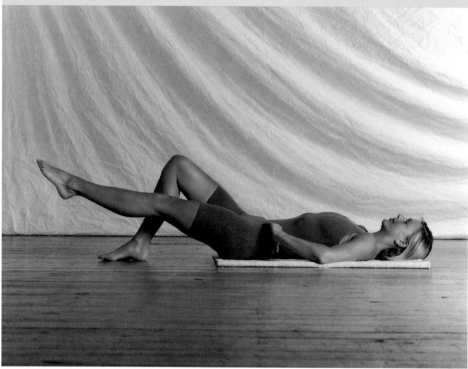

Run-through

Stand facing a wall, with your hands placed on the wall at shoulder level, squeezing your buttock muscles and tightening your low abdominal muscles. Slowly lift your right leg from the hip, keeping your hip, knee, and foot in line, until it is bent at right angles from the hip. Hold this position for 20 seconds. Repeat three times on each leg.

Leg raise

Lying on your back, with your right knee bent and right foot flat on the floor, tighten your lower abdominal muscles and keep your lower back stable, neither arching nor flattening it. With your left knee straight and toes pointing, slowly lift your left leg slightly off the floor. Hold this position for 10 seconds before slowly relaxing and repeating on the other leg. Do this exercise 10 times on each leg.

Seated crease

Sitting in a chair, straighten your back so you lift up your chest, and tighten your low abdominal muscles. Slowly lift your right leg from the hip, bringing your knee slightly toward you and keeping it bent at the same angle. All the movement should come from your right side – don't use your left leg to push, and don't lean to the left. Hold this position for 15 seconds, before relaxing and repeat six times on each leg.

Routines

It is not difficult to fit regular exercise into your day-to-day life, especially when you do not have to devote a long block of time to it. Here are some exercises that take only a few minutes and are tailored for different circumstances.

Pause gymnastics are exercises designed to be done every half-hour when you are working at a desk. They will help you to avoid the stiffness and strain that comes from a sedentary lifestyle.

Home energizers are perfect for people who do not play sports or go to fitness classes, but want to stretch and tone the body through exercises at home.

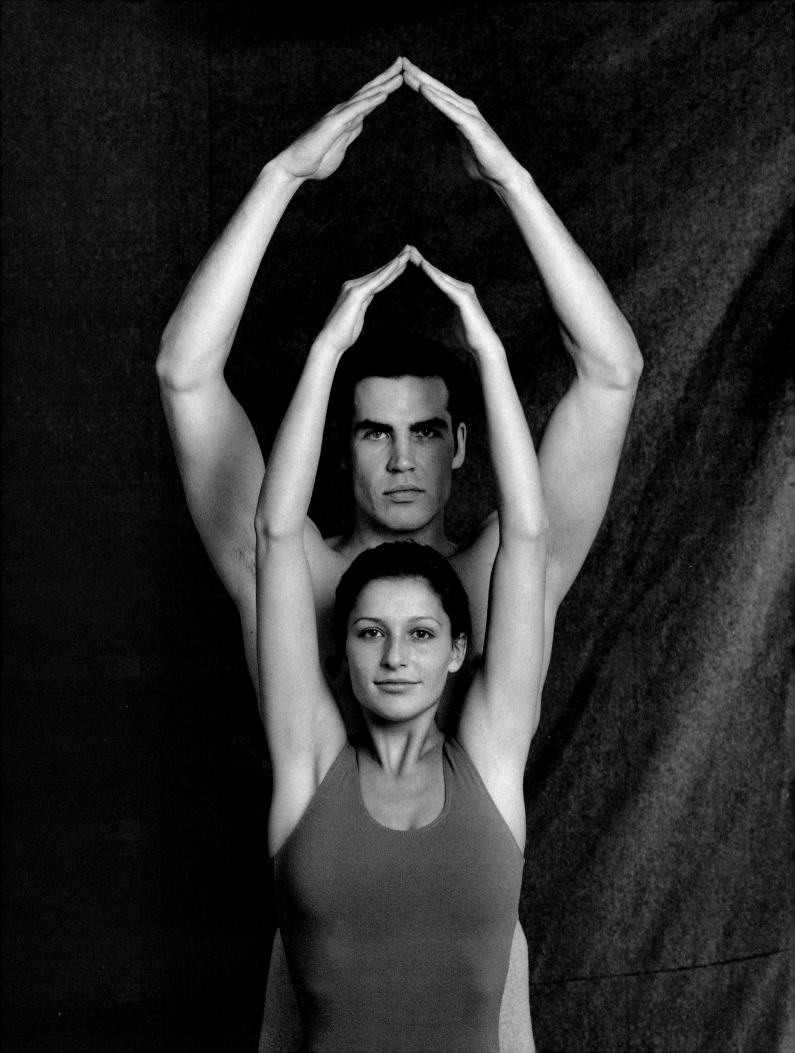

Pause gymnastics

Choose two or three of the following exercises to do every half-hour when you are sitting at a desk or working at a keyboard. They will fend off the stiffness that comes from sitting at a desk all day and will improve your postural awareness. The stretches for your forearms and hands will also keep your wrist joints flexible and the tendons in your forearms and wrists supple. These are familiar problem areas for people who work on keyboards or do repetitive tasks during the day.

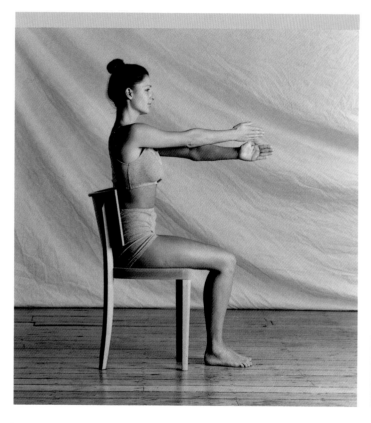

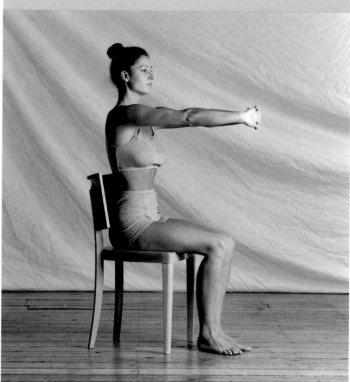

Shoulder stretch

Sit tall, lifting a little at your chest. Reach out in front with both your arms, with your elbows and wrists straight and keeping your shoulder blades tucked back and down. Slowly cross your arms from the shoulders until you feel a stretch in both shoulders.

When you feel the stretch, hold the position for 10 seconds. Relax and repeat three times. This is a good stretch for the muscles at the top of your shoulders, which tend to tighten if you sit at your desk for long periods of time.

Palm pull

This exercise will stretch your wrist and elbow joints as well as the tendons in your forearms. Sit tall, lifting a little at your chest. Reach straight out in front of you from your shoulders, and interlace your fingers so your palms are facing toward you, then turn your palms away at the wrist. Stretch your arms forward from your shoulders. Hold this position for six seconds then relax and repeat twice. Make sure you keep a good upper back position as you do this exercise.

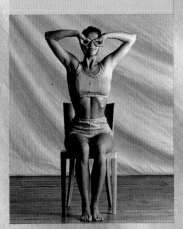

Mr Magoo

This funny position will stretch your upper arms and forearms. Sitting tall and lifting a little at your chest, make circles with the thumb and index finger of both hands. This is the tricky part: turn your palms up and over toward your face, with your fingers pointing down and resting along the side of your face, so the circles you made with your thumb and index finger fit around your eyes like glasses. Lift your elbows to stretch your arms slightly behind you. Hold this stretch for three seconds and repeat three times.

Wrestler hold

Sitting tall and lifting a little at your chest, reach with your right hand around your back and up in between your shoulder blades. Reach as far as you can, feeling a stretch at the front of your shoulder and in between your shoulder blades. Hold this stretch for three seconds before relaxing and repeating three times on each arm.

❶

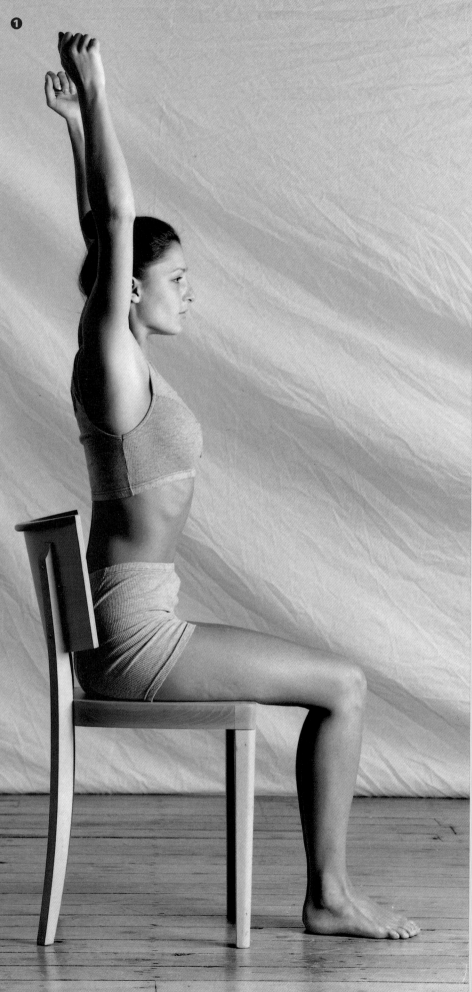

❷

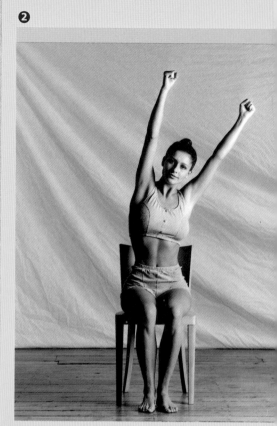

Arm extender

This exercise will loosen your upper back and your arms.

Sitting tall and lifting a little at your chest, make fists and reach with both of your arms above your head (1). Your shoulders, elbows, and hands should be straight above you. Reach a little higher with your right hand, and then with your left. Repeat this exercise three times on each arm.

You can vary this position so it stretches your entire spine – this variation is ideal after you have been sitting for a long time. With your arms straight above you, bend sideways, starting the movement from low down your torso, keeping both buttocks on the chair and your chest facing forward (2). Repeat three times on each side.

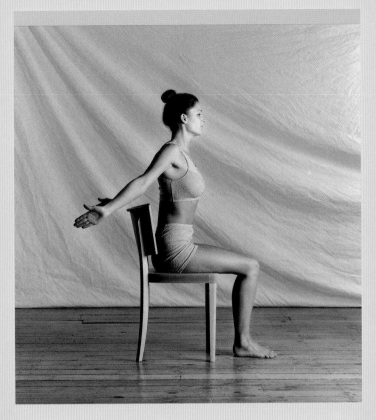

Airplane
Sitting tall, lift a little at your chest and rotate your hands so your palms face the ceiling, your thumbs pointing behind you. Raise your arms, keeping them straight, and draw them gently behind your back. Hold your arms out straight like wings, maintaining the stretch for six seconds. Repeat this exercise three times.

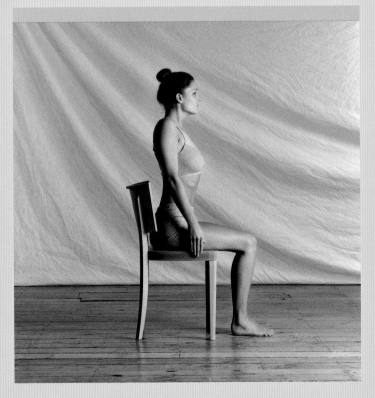

Seated shoulder circle
This exercise will help you to relax your upper back and free your shoulders. Sit tall in your chair, lifting a little at your chest. Shrug your shoulders up toward your ears and then roll them backward, making sure the movement is coming from your shoulders. Repeat this circular movement six times. Relax the shoulder muscles as you let go of each circle.

Home energizers

These exercises are specifically designed for people who do not play sports or participate in any other fitness activities, but who are looking for simple, effective exercises that that stretch and tone the whole body. You don't even have to do them all at once. They take only a few seconds each, so they are can easily be incorporated into your day-to-day life. Try doing a few during the commercial breaks of your favorite TV program or when you take a break from reading or preparing something to eat.

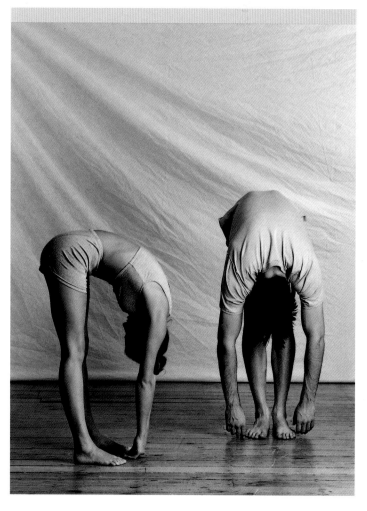

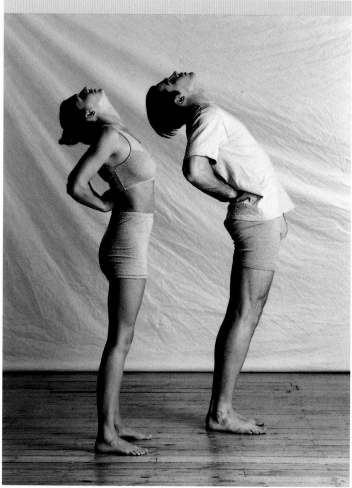

The puppet
Imagine yourself suspended by strings like a puppet. Think how it would feel if the strings supporting the top of your body broke.

Stand with your weight equally over both feet. Starting with your head, curl forward so your chin touches your chest, then continue the curling movement from your upper back down. Relax totally into the stretch for 10 seconds. On the way back up, gently uncurl from your lower back to your upper back, then your neck and head.

Standing cobra
Stand with your weight equally through both of your legs and knees straight but not locked. Make fists with your hands and place them in the small of your back, and tuck your elbows behind you. Keep your head facing to the front as you arch back over your fists. Hold this stretch for six seconds before relaxing and repeating three times. Don't push this stretch too far, especially if you have a weak lower back. When your back is supple, you can include your head in the backward bend.

Simon says
Standing with your weight equally over both feet and your knees straight, place your hands on your head, and without twisting from your waist, bend to the side so your left shoulder moves toward your left hip. Don't push too far – you should feel a gentle stretch in your back. Return to the starting position, then repeat on the other side. Repeat slowly and gently four times on each side.

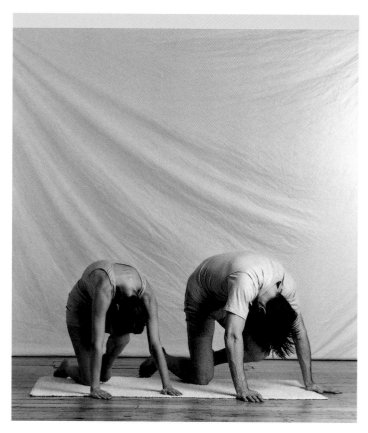

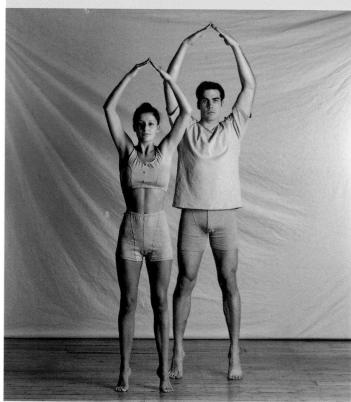

Advanced crawl

Begin on your hands and knees on the floor, with your back and neck straight. Bend your left knee up toward your chest, and as you do, tuck your chin down toward your chest, curling your back. Keep your weight balanced through both of your hands and your right knee.

Repeat this exercise six times on each leg. This will improve the suppleness of your whole spine.

Ballet dancer

This is a good exercise for your upper back, buttocks, and low abdominal muscles.

Standing with your weight on the balls of your feet, raise yourself onto your toes, maintaining your balance. As you breathe in deeply, raise both arms out to the side and up so that your hands touch above your head. Slowly breathe out as you lower yourself onto flat feet and allow your arms to return to your sides. Take your time, concentrating on your balance, and try to reach as high as you can.

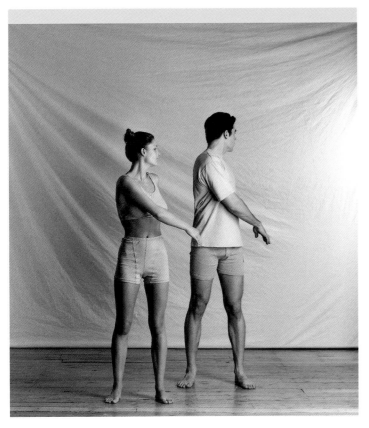

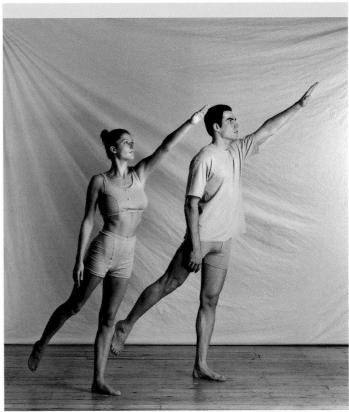

Pinwheel

Stand with your weight equally over both feet and your knees slightly bent. Twist your head, shoulders, and trunk to the left, then return to the starting position before twisting to the other side. Repeat six times on each side. This is a good stretch for your spine, but it also works the muscles of your back, neck, and shoulders.

Diagonal reach

Stand, balancing with most of your weight on your left leg. Concentrating on maintaining your balance, reach forward and up with your left arm and raise your right leg behind you. You can place your left arm lightly on a wall for balance. Repeat this movement three times with your left arm and right leg, then three times for the right arm and left leg.

This exercise will improve the flexibility of your spine, shoulder, and hip joints. It will also tone the muscles of your buttocks, stomach, and upper back.

Index

Acknowledgments

Illustrations: Marks Creative

Additional text: Sara Black

Indexer: Clare Richards

Proofreader: Phyllida Hancock

Chair: Montego, by Habitat

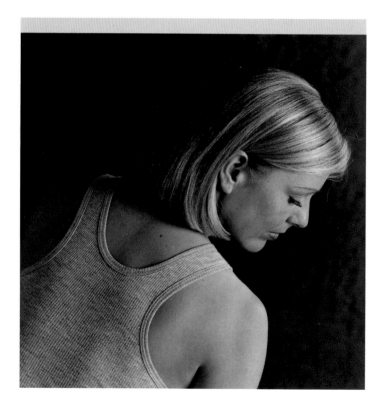